The Complete

Spa Manual
for Homeowners:

A Step-by-Step Maintenance and Therapy Guide

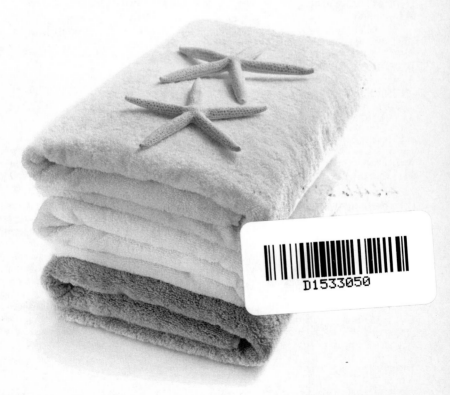

By Dan Hardy

With Foreword By Daniel Harrison

THE COMPLETE SPA MANUAL FOR HOMEOWNERS: A STEP-BY-STEP
MAINTENANCE AND THERAPY GUIDE

Copyright © 2011 Atlantic Publishing Group, Inc.
1405 SW 6th Avenue • Ocala, Florida 34471 • Phone 800-814-1132 • Fax 352-622-1875
Web site: www.atlantic-pub.com • E-mail: sales@atlantic-pub.com
SAN Number: 268-1250

Library of Congress Cataloging-in-Publication Data

Hardy, Dan, 1953-
  The complete spa manual for homeowners : a step-by-step maintenance and therapy guide /
by Dan Hardy.
    p. cm.
  Includes bibliographical references and index.
  ISBN-13: 978-1-60138-263-4 (alk. paper)
  ISBN-10: 1-60138-263-4 (alk. paper)
  1. Hot tubs. 2. Spa pools. I. Title.
  TH6501.H37 2010
  690'.896--dc22

                                    2010011611

4646 5091 8/11

Printed in the United States

PROJECT MANAGER: Shannon McCarthy
PEER REVIEWER: Marilee Griffin
PHOTO EDITING & ILLUSTRATIONS: Harrison Kuo
INTERIOR DESIGN: Samantha Martin
FRONT & BACK COVER DESIGN: Jackie Miller • millerjackiej@gmail.com

Printed on Recycled Paper

We recently lost our beloved pet "Bear," who was not only our best and dearest friend but also the "Vice President of Sunshine" here at Atlantic Publishing. He did not receive a salary but worked tirelessly 24 hours a day to please his parents. Bear was a rescue dog that turned around and showered myself, my wife, Sherri, his grandparents Jean, Bob, and Nancy, and every person and animal he met (maybe not rabbits) with friendship and love. He made a lot of people smile every day.

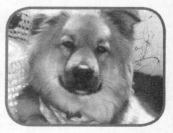

We wanted you to know that a portion of the profits of this book will be donated to The Humane Society of the United States. –*Douglas & Sherri Brown*

The human-animal bond is as old as human history. We cherish our animal companions for their unconditional affection and acceptance. We feel a thrill when we glimpse wild creatures in their natural habitat or in our own backyard.

Unfortunately, the human-animal bond has at times been weakened. Humans have exploited some animal species to the point of extinction.

The Humane Society of the United States makes a difference in the lives of animals here at home and worldwide. The HSUS is dedicated to creating a world where our relationship with animals is guided by compassion. We seek a truly humane society in which animals are respected for their intrinsic value, and where the human-animal bond is strong.

Want to help animals? We have plenty of suggestions. Adopt a pet from a local shelter, join The Humane Society and be a part of our work to help companion animals and wildlife. You will be funding our educational, legislative, investigative and outreach projects in the U.S. and across the globe.

Or perhaps you'd like to make a memorial donation in honor of a pet, friend or relative? You can through our Kindred Spirits program. And if you'd like to contribute in a more structured way, our Planned Giving Office has suggestions about estate planning, annuities, and even gifts of stock that avoid capital gains taxes.

Maybe you have land that you would like to preserve as a lasting habitat for wildlife. Our Wildlife Land Trust can help you. Perhaps the land you want to share is a backyard— that's enough. Our Urban Wildlife Sanctuary Program will show you how to create a habitat for your wild neighbors.

So you see, it's easy to help animals. And The HSUS is here to help.

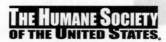

2100 L Street NW • Washington, DC 20037 • 202-452-1100
www.hsus.org

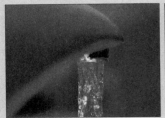 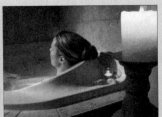 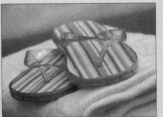

Acknowledgements: *I would like to thank the owner of Premium Leisure, Brian Wiley, for allowing me to invade their factory and take pictures of their operation as well as obtain information to help produce this book. The information that was provided was extremely valuable and let me see some of the newest and best ways to build a spa as well as the new equipment being used. The team that I was fortunate enough to watch in their daily job was a very professional group and showed a strong desire to produce an excellent product.*

I would like to thank Tammie Colombotti for her help in making arrangements for my invasion of the Premium Leisure plant in St. Petersburg, Florida. Tammie is in sales and is a very knowledge-able individual on their product, and she was most helpful to me.

TABLE OF CONTENTS

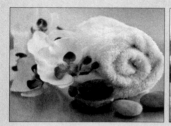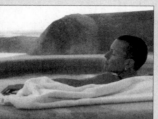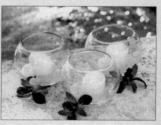

Chapter 3: Spa Plumbing 91

Chapter 4: Water Chemistry 101

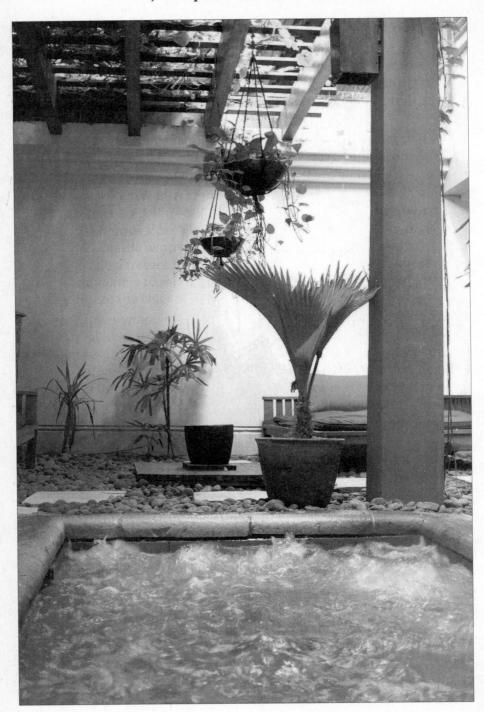

FOREWORD

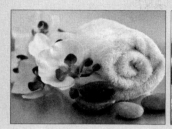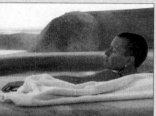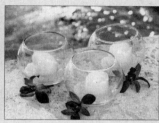

It was a cold, clear night in 1982 and I had just finished a long day of skiing at Vermont's Okemo Mountain. I had traveled up from New York with some friends who had arranged our lodging in a quaint New England bed and breakfast. Unbeknownst to me, the facility had a small indoor pool, a sauna, and a hot tub tucked away in a back basement room.

"Hey, does anyone want to go jump in the hot tub?" my friend asked, his eyes gleeful.

"Sure," I said, not quite certain what I was agreeing to at that point. We gathered up the girls and took a trip down to the hot tub room.

In 1982, hot tubs and spas were not very commonplace. Hotels, health clubs, and resorts tended to be the exclusive domain of the hot tub. I had actually never seen one in person at that point, and as far as I was concerned, they only really existed in movies or on television. Visions of Jerry Garcia lookalikes soaking in round, outdoor wooden tubs in the forests of California filled my mind.

"What am I in for?" I thought to myself. "Is this going to be like some sleazy movie? Am I going to get a disease?" I did not want to sit in murky green water with other people.

When we got to the pool area, I began to feel a little better once I saw that everything appeared nice and clean. "Come on, let's go in the sauna first," my girlfriend suggested.

We all stuffed ourselves into the tiny sauna. At first, it was pretty hot and uncomfortable, but my muscles had been aching from that first-day-of-the-season ski expedition, and the dry, hot air was oddly compelling.

After a few minutes in the sauna, my friend said we should go out and jump in the swimming pool now that we were all very hot from our sauna experience. My friend yelled out; "This is either going to feel great, or it's going to kill you!"

We all boldly filed out of the sauna and jumped into the ice-cold — albeit crisp — indoor pool.

"Wow!" my girlfriend, who went first, yelled as we saw her emerge like a rocket from the water. "That feels great."

I thought she was nuts, but I followed suit and took the plunge myself. The sudden shock from dry heat to freezing water was invigorating, to say the least. It was considerably more enjoyable than I had ever thought it would have been. I could feel all the blood in my veins pumping as I swam around the pool for a minute or so, waiting for my poor body to acclimate to the abrupt temperature change. Not another minute went by when my friend yelled out, "Now, everybody out of the pool and into the hot tub!"

"What?" I thought. "You have to be kidding me!"

With great trepidation, the rest of us, fairly invigorated by the somewhat unusual experience at that point, followed him like lemmings into the hot tub room. Obviously, he had done this whole routine before and knew that as crazy as it sounded, our little band of skiers would ultimately be quite satisfied with our unusual holiday jaunt. We were experiencing cardiovascular hydrotherapy at its best, although none of us realized it at that point in time.

Once inside the hot tub room, most of my existing fears started to subside — it was tastefully designed with a large fiberglass octagon-shaped hot tub in the middle of the room. The room had cedar planking on the walls with mirrors set into the wood, alternating with the planks. Combined with the amber light emanating from the clear, warm, bubbling water of the tub, the whole ambiance of the room was very relaxing and quite womb-like. "Now this is something I think I'll really like," I thought.

I entered the hot tub and immediately felt at home. In direct juxtaposition to jarring experience with the sauna and the swimming pool, this tub gave me a feeling of warm, cozy comfort. As I enjoyed the swirling waters pulsating out of the spa jets that eased my aching muscles, all the stress and tension of a rather long and arduous day disappeared. I seemed to enter my own little relaxing world. While all my friends were sprawling out and joking in the tub, I can clearly remember being quiet. I was having one of those moments of clarity you only hear about others having. I did not fully realize how that moment was about to change my life forever.

"Wow — I bet people on Long Island would really like this," I said to my friends, who seemed like they could care less at that moment. "I wonder if I could sell these things?"

"I don't know," my girlfriend said. "Why are you always thinking about business? Why don't you just chill out and enjoy yourself for once?"

Well, anyone who knows me will understand how hard it is for me to truly relax. And while being in the hot tub was certainly one of the closest things to nirvana I had ever experienced up to that point in my life, the little gears in my mind were in full swing, pondering how this experience could be brought to the masses and how I could find out more about this magical, mysterious thing that had somehow been kept off my radar for so long.

Needless to say, we were in that hot tub more than we were on the ski slopes that weekend — and I was truly moved by the experience. I had never felt so relaxed, so invigorated, and so rested all at the same time.

"I have to look into this further," I told my girlfriend as we packed our belongings and got ready for our long, cold, icy ride back to New York.

Over the next few months, I investigated everything I could about the state-of-the-art hot tub industry, if you could even call it that. In 1982, there really was not much of a hot tub industry at all. There were only a few companies nationwide that were making what you would remotely recognize as the hot tub spas of today.

I was introduced to Artie Jost of AJ Spas in early 1983. Artie had a similar interest in hot tubs and opened up a small hot tub manufacturing shop out of the back of an appliance store in Patchogue on Long Island. Soon after receiving quite an education from Artie, I opened Long Island Hot Tubs, one of the first all hot tub spa stores in the United States.

I can remember the first home improvement show where we exhibited hot tubs to the public. It was in a shopping mall on Long Island's North Shore area, known for its high-end homes and old-money mansions. We brought an old, rickety fiberglass spa to the show and were virtually inundated with requests for more information about the portable spa, this relatively new and unique invention. Prior to this, most people, even the rich and famous, only saw or got to use hot tub spas in health clubs, gyms, hotels, or resorts.

"What is this, one of them new-fangled 'Sacuzzi's?'" we were asked repeatedly as the initial wave of consumers got their first taste of hot tubs for the home. From the response, we could see that this was something that was going to catch on in a big way. We were very surprised — and happy — to have sold 21 tubs during that first home improvement show.

As the popularity of the residential hot tub caught on during the latter half of the 1980s, we saw an influx of new spa brands becoming available almost on a monthly basis. Companies like Hot Spring® Spas, Sundance®, Hawkeye Spas®, Baja Spas®, Regency, Nemco, and Jacuzzi® became commonplace names in the new lexicon of the late 1980s Reagan era of self-indulgence.

As the demand for hot tubs grew and the money started pouring into our little industry, natural capitalistic innovations rapidly took place, greatly improving and standardizing the portable spa. Technological advances in acrylic vacuum-forming machines made the complicated designs and seating patterns of the tubs commonplace. Circuit boards made the **spa packs** — the control system or brains of the hot tub — ever more able to control multiple jet pumps, air bubblers, heaters, and even color-changing mood-lighting systems, which all converged to increase the visual appeal and functionality of the hot tub to the end user.

However, there was a dirty little secret brewing within the industry. Although consumers were truly enjoying the daily use of their home hot tub units, many of them were complaining to their dealers about the care and maintenance necessary to keep their hot tub water clear, sanitary, and smelling fresh. The amount of time and money it took to properly maintain a residential hot tub unit was threatening the very existence and stability of the fledgling hot tub industry.

I heard it almost on a daily basis from consumers: "You sold this to me and I can't keep it clean."

"My wife got an infection from using your spa."

"I am going to go broke with all the chlorine and chemicals that I have to add to my spa on a daily basis. What are you going to do about it?"

This was rapidly becoming a concern among spa dealers and manufacturers, as the number of installed units nationwide grew to more than 1 million. Something had to be done — and fast.

Luckily, by the late 1980s, there was a plethora of new chemicals and sanitizing devices that made hot tub maintenance considerably easier. Bromine, ozone, and a host of alternative, eco-friendly spa-water sanitizers quickly flooded the market, and their success spread like wildfire among the hot tub community.

Nowadays, anyone can wake up in the morning and decide they want a hot tub in their home. They can look up a few brands on the Internet, find a local dealer, and, in many cases, have their very own portable hot tub spa delivered to their house to use that night. And with all the new technology, many spa brands even offer built-in stereos, waterproof flat screen TVs, LED color-changing mood lighting, waterfalls, and other exotic features to add to your relaxing hot tub experience.

But as with anything, you should research thoroughly before purchasing. Just like cars and computers, the hot tubs of today do need some periodic maintenance that you will have to learn about after you start using your tub.

In his new book, *The Complete Spa Manual for Homeowners*, industry veteran Dan Hardy covers absolutely everything you should know before you select a hot tub spa for your home. He also covers, in great detail, the dos and don'ts of hot tub care and maintenance. Hardy has gone through great lengths to sift through all the information out there and presents it all to you in an understandable, fun-to-read format for the average hot tub buyer or owner.

One thing is for sure — the relaxation and hydrotherapy you can get from owning your own hot tub spa is quite remarkable. This one little invention will help you feel better, sleep easier, and provide a focal point for interaction with family and friends for years to come.

There are few things in life that can provide you with the daily rejuvenation a hot tub provides. I wish you all the best with your spa, and I sincerely thank Dan Hardy for his efforts in educating the public about our industry's wonderful products.

And as I always say at the end of my **Poolandspa.TV** videos and TV shows, "Happy tubbing."

DANIEL HARRISON

President

Poolandspa.com

Poolandspa.TV

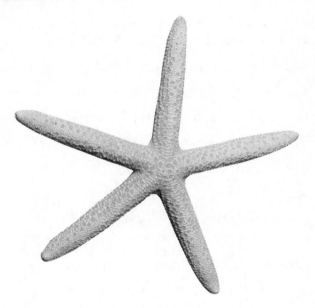

INTRODUCTION

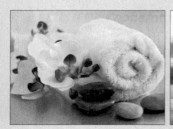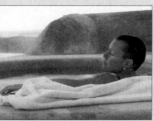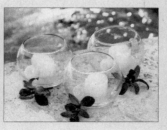

and History

F or thousands of years, man has used hot water to soothe old bones. Some ancient people used the watering holes for rituals, some of which included animal or human sacrifices.

About 4,000 years ago, the Egyptians used hot therapeutic baths on a regular basis for enjoyment and healing. History says that around 600 B.C., a Persian king named Phraortes had a hot tub carved out of a large piece of granite. Plato, Homer, and Hippocrates used these hot water pools for their personal enjoyment and rituals. They realized their therapeutic possibilities. The Greeks often used hot tubs for social events and had public bathing establishments.

The Emperor Agrippa of Rome built one of the first man-made, large-scale spas, which were usually called **thermae**. As rulers normally do, each subsequent emperor tried to outdo the last in these great places they enjoyed. They used these spas to help heal war wounds and aching bodies and were used to help heal digestive disorders, lung disorders, infections, and heart-related problems that we know as hypertension. In order to outdo each other, some rulers even had restaurants, massage parlors, and brothels built with their spas. Back then, it was all about pleasure, so it was not uncommon to have a complete package of entertainment in one location.

Simply placing rocks in a fire and adding the hot rocks into the water, which transferred the heat from the stones to the water, heated the pools. Some pools and spas were built using water from natural hot springs. Some of the Romans were able to build spas that had natural filtration systems by using a pit where debris could fall and allowing clean water to flow into the spa.

The Greeks had hot baths around 500 B.C. that were built near volcanoes and hot springs, allowing them to use the natural hot mineral water. This method was easier than heating rocks. The Greeks, like the Romans, also had large public hot tubs, and some had buildings with private rooms and even steam rooms.

Between 460 and 375 B.C., the founder of medicine, Hippocrates, used the hot water tubs to treat rheumatism (pain in the muscles, joints, tendons, and bones) and jaundice (the yellowing of the skin and sometimes eyes). This was the first of what we call **hydrotherapy**, which is a treatment that uses water to either internally or externally to treat medical conditions. It was so important to them that Plato claimed that if a person could not swim, then he or she was uneducated.

The word "spa" came from the Hungarian word of "spa," which referred to the natural mineral springs. In the English town of Bath, the spas were used from 800 B.C. and continue to be used today. Even Queen Elizabeth I used them. They were 120°F, could generate up to 1 million gallons of mineral water per day, and contained more than 30 elements, including calcium, sulfur, potassium, and magnesium. The water even had a slight radioactive reading, according to historians.

In Japan, they have a saying: "Mizu no kokoro." It simply means, "mind like water." This refers to the peaceful state of being in harmony with all things on earth. As we have seen reflected in many old movies, public bathing facilities have been commonplace in Japan for many years. It was common in Japan in the older days for everyone to bathe together, and warm water massage was also a common practice.

Our military personnel who fought overseas brought this idea back to America in great force after World War II. However, it was not the first time hot water bathing and healing were used in the United States. In the early 1700s, many communities enjoyed hot water entertainment. In Saratoga, New York, the High Rock Spring was first used by Native Americans. It was rumored that in the late 1700s, British patriot Sir William Johnson was ailing of a bad medical problem and was carried to this place for a cure. General Philip Schuyler, George Washington, and Alexander Hamilton also used this facility for numerous purposes.

President Franklin D. Roosevelt had a home in Warm Springs, Colorado, that he called his "Little White House." During his administration from 1933 to 1945, he used the hot water therapy there to help the pain his polio caused. He later dedicated the facility to people with disabilities.

Across the United States, these bathing facilities were used by many types of people for numerous reasons — enjoyment being high on the list. Around 1958, hot tubs made out of wood started to become popular in California. The first of these were made from old wine barrels. They were soon built larger for the social status of owning one afforded.

Today, hot tubs and spas are a multi-million dollar industry. They can be found in health spas, sports locker rooms, motels, cruise ships, and just about anywhere that provides health, fitness, and entertainment. Most of all, they are becoming extremely common in the households; that is where this book, which is geared toward families looking to purchase a spa or hot tub for personal use (or for those who already have one), comes in.

I started working with electricity at an early age in the automotive field. Cars and trucks use direct current instead of alternating current, which is used for residential and commercial needs. What I learned is that electricity does the same thing no matter the voltage. Residential electricity is easier to repair and install than automotive electrical, which is why spa repair came easy to me if I had a diagram or an electrical schematic for guidance. Understanding flows and hydraulics is the hard part. How the water flows is, in my opinion, at the heart of a good spa.

Taking care of your spa is part of taking care of your family. It can be a very useful thing to have, or it can be a monster that drives you crazy and can be unhealthy. Learning to take care of your spa properly will ensure you and your family will have a safe and enjoyable spa experience. This book was designed to help you pick out your spa, maintain it, and enjoy it. It is geared to the spa owner and not the professional. I hope that it will be of great use to you.

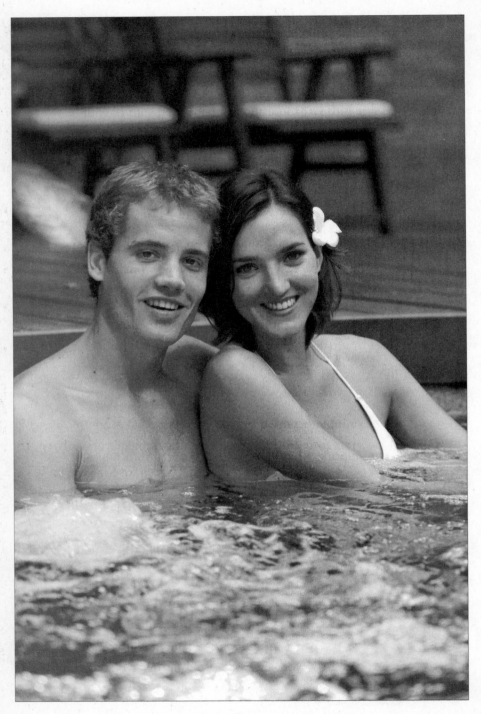

CHAPTER ONE

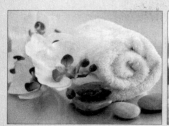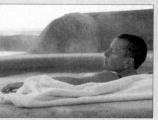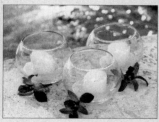

What Are You Looking For?

B efore we start talking about what you would like in a spa, let us talk about maintenance. If you expect a spa to take care of itself, then do not buy one. A heated spa is a natural place for bacteria to grow, and not only can this be dangerous, but some people have died from problems resulting from using a spa. *This will be covered in more detail in Chapter 4*, but if you have no intent on taking care of your spa and spending some time performing general upkeep and maintenance, then you should seriously reconsider purchasing a spa.

When you make up your mind to purchase a spa or hot tub, you need to sit down and figure out exactly what you are looking for. The questions you need to ask yourself or your family are as follows:

- What function do you want a spa or hot tub to perform? Are you looking for some therapy function or do you just want to sit in warm water? Is there a particular part of your body you would like to treat for pain? Are you just looking for relaxation and stress relief? Or is it just going to be a toy that you brag to your friends about?

- How much are you willing to pay for a spa or hot tub? Price determines what systems you can get and what functions a hot tub or spa can perform. Are maintenance costs and operational cost an issue?

- How often do you plan to use the equipment?

A hot tub can be made of different products, from vinyl to fiberglass. It has hot water and some type of circulation and water filtration system. These are usually basic systems with not much of a technical function. The fewer functions and less equipment a hot tub includes, the less it should cost.

A spa, on the other hand, should circulate and heat water. I call a spa a device that is totally self-contained. These should be able to heat water, deliver therapeutic comfort, filter out unwanted particles from the water, and sanitize and kill bacteria. It should have various functions to perform a therapeutic action. Spas can hold one or many people. Now, when I discuss spas, I am talking about the ones that usually are portable and not the pool and spa combinations. The combos usually are very limited in their therapeutic functions, and it is better to describe them as entertainment spas.

In a pool and spa combination, usually the equipment consists of a heater, a circulation pump, and perhaps a blower. These blowers force air into the spa, either through some type of hole in the spa or through jets that mix the water and air together. Seating is usually just a bench, and you can adjust your position to have water flow on a certain part of your body. Most combinations do a good job if designed properly, but they are considered inferior in regard to their special functions. With a portable spa, you can get jet packs and flexible jets that can be directed to massage different parts of your body, and these jets could not be installed in a concrete pool/spa combination. In addition, these pool/spa combos usually cost much more to build.

Some portable spas come with water circulators that offer limited functions and only circulate water to give the impression that some therapeutic value is being performed. Other than the stress relief that one gets from warm water, which is very healthy, they cannot do anything other than just circulate water and can be purchased sometimes for less than $1,000. A true spa is one that has various seating positions and jets for different functions that are designed to work on a particular part of the body. Spas can provide numerous health benefits that will be discussed later in this chapter.

The use of alcohol in a hot tub must be limited. Drinking and sitting in hot water can be a dangerous thing. Both alcohol and sitting in hot water expands your blood vessels, which increases your body temperature. The use of any medications should be discussed with your doctor to make sure that sitting in hot water will not interact with any drugs that you are taking. Excessive drinking and the relaxation that hot water provides may cause you to pass out in the spa. Caution and common sense must be used in a hot tub or spa.

The average time for soaking in a hot tub or spa is between 10 and 15 minutes at a temperature of 98° to 104°F. If you have just purchase a spa, limit your time and lower the water temperature to find what is comfortable for you. Pregnant women should not use a hot tub or spa unless cleared by their doctor. According to the Association of Pool and Spa Professionals, pregnant women are especially sensitive to high temperatures, and spending too much time in a hot tub can elevate body temperature and the temperature of internal organs beyond what is considered safe for both the mother and the baby.

When I was younger and had less sense, I used my dad's hot tub with a friend when he was out of town. He kept the temperature at 102°F, and after about 40 minutes of sitting in the hot tub, I was going to get another drink but physically could not get out of the tub. My legs did not work nor did anything else want to function; I had to be pulled out of the spa. I can say that I slept a long time and in a deep sleep that night, but at least I was able to wake up the next morning. Some have not had that luxury and have collapsed and drowned in their spa. The reason this happens is that the muscles, when hot, push the blood toward the skin so that the body can sweat out the excessive temperature; this weakens the muscles due to blood loss. Since the body cannot sweat out the heat while in hot water, the muscles continue to drain themselves of the blood, which in turn saps your strength. Make sure you are responsible when you are using your spa. You should also never leave children in a spa for long periods and never leave them unsupervised.

Health Benefits

One of the greatest things about owning your own spa is the ability to use it for health reasons. Some can offer health benefits including aromatherapy, hydrotherapy, and reflexology. There are many documented health benefits to using a spa:

- **Hydrotherapy** is sometimes called massage because it performs the same function. Hydrotherapy first relaxes the individual and slows down a busy day and calms the user. It relieves nerves that have pressure on them from sore muscles or tension. One of the main functions of a good spa is stress relief. It relaxes the user, and, depending on the individual, he or she is able to get a good night's sleep after enjoying the spa.

- **Aromatherapy** refers to treatment using special scents. These scents are absorbed through the body, either by breathing them in or by absorbing them through the skin into the bloodstream. This form of holistic treatment is one of the fastest-growing fields in alternative medicine.

- **Reflexology** is the therapeutic method of applying deep pressure to reflex points in the hands and feet. The theory is that this pressure affects other parts of the body. Actual human body maps have been produced to show certain areas in the feet or hands that affect different muscles, organs, and functions. It can also be referred to as water acupuncture and to top it off, it really works!

Some critics may look at all of the people who utilize these therapies and say all they want is to sit in hot water and enjoy a beer. A person has to believe that these therapies are beneficial and will work for them. After all, most have been proven for thousands of years.

Medical opinions of the use of hot water vary. I have been told by people in the hydrotherapy field that the use of hot water and even a sauna can cause the human body to produce more white blood cells and aid in the building of antibodies. (White blood cells are what fight infections.) As your body temperature rises, sitting in hot water makes your body think it has some infection so the white cell count goes up to help fight the infection. In some ways, this is good, and in others, it can be bad. Consulting your doctor before starting any therapy regimen is always recommended.

In the *Miller-Keane Medical Dictionary, 2000,* it explains that physicians and physical therapists do recommend the use of water therapy and massage as a form of rehabilitative therapy. The Arthritis Foundation believes the massage effect and buoyancy of water is needed to not only exercise the joints but also relax muscles.

The Arthritis Foundation states that exercise in water leads to mood changes and actually enhances the sense of self-esteem and accomplishment. Heat dilates your blood vessels, which increases the flow of blood to injured tissues of your body and may accelerate the healing process. Hot water can reduce pain by stimulating the release of endorphins.

Exercising in a spa lets your body limit the weight bearing on your joints. It is said that when you are submersed in water, your body's weight is reduced by 90 percent. This lets you exercise your muscles while limiting the damage done to strained joints and muscles. It also relieves the tension often related to stress that can cause physical problems.

Research has suggested that a spa can aid in weight loss. When you are in hot water, your heart rate increases, but at the same time, the water lowers your blood pressure. This allows you to increase your heart rate without the stress put on the heart. There are claims a spa can help you lose weight and reduce cellulite because soaking in a hot tub simulates exercise, dilating the blood vessels and promoting better circulation.

When a person is under stress, the heart works harder. For some people, breathing can become more rapid and shallow, and the digestive system can slow down. The Centers for Disease Control and Prevention has estimated that 80 percent of all diseases are stress-related; this in itself is a reason to own a spa, or at least use one. The endorphins that are released while in a hot-water environment will relieve the stress in your life. It is up to you to get rid of the stress that you have.

In 1999, the *New England Journal of Medicine* published an article that claimed soaking in hot water for 30 minutes a day can help people suffering from type 2 diabetes reduce their blood sugar levels and improve sleep for patients. Again, people suffering from type 2 diabetes should always consult with their doctor before starting a new health care regime.

For those who are really interested in the health benefits of hot water, you should research further to see if using any of these techniques can be a benefit or a problem when using a spa. Always remember to start slow; begin with a lower temperature and less time to see what you prefer and how your body reacts. After you have been using the spa for a while, you can then adjust time and temperature to suit your preferences. *There is more health information in Chapter 6.*

Patio Design

For those of you who want to spruce up your patio area, a spa is a good item to do it with. Spas can incorporate decks around them that are raised, or you can even sink the spa into the deck. An area that a spa is located in can be landscaped with flowers and scrubs and all kinds of vegetation to make it look like a tropical paradise. Gazebos have been used to cover a spa to provide a nice look or to protect the spa and the bather from weather. Sitting in a spa under some kind of protective cover is a nice experience during a rainstorm or even when it is snowing. Care must be taken to not be in the spa when there is lightning in the immediate area.

An outdoor spa with a screened-in porch is great to help eliminate the different insects that may swarm you while you are in the spa. A screened enclosure keeps debris such as leaves and other things that fly in the air away from the spa. This helps you keep a clean area where you can enjoy your experience and not have to spend excess time cleaning.

The important thing to remember when you are designing an area of entertainment using your spa is that you need to leave the spa panels exposed for inspections and repairs. The spa needs to be located so that you will notice if there is a leak from the underside of the shell. All your work designing and maintaining an area will be in vain if you have to dismantle what you have built to repair some small leak or replace a defective part. This problem occurs often when a designer can make your backyard beautiful but has no idea about what is required to maintain a spa. This is a thought for you to remember when you plan your backyard.

Also note that some landscapers and designers may not know that the mist that comes off a spa can damage or kill certain plants. When foliage is close to the water of a spa or pool, it can make a homeowner very upset to see expensive plants deteriorate. Care must be taken when choosing plants and deciding where you will put them.

CASE STUDY: SPA OWNERS DAVE AND ROSE WERTHEIM

Dave Wertheim
Roseville, California

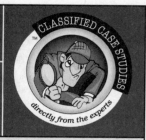

We have purchased two spas over the years: the first was purchased in 1984, and the spa we have now was purchased in 2004 for around $7,500. We went to several retail outlets and home shows, but each time we purchased our spas from friends in the industry.

We love enjoying the jets in our spa after our children have gone to bed for the evening. It is a great way to enjoy quality time with each other and review our day. When we first purchased our spa, we used it almost every day, sometimes before work and then again at night. Now we use it once or twice a week. We primarily use the spa for therapeutic purposes after a hard workout as well as a getaway to spend some time together.

Maintenance is very important to keep the spa running efficiently. We check the bromine levels and alkalinity twice a week; clean the filters once a week; clean suction ports and drains as needed when the jet pressure is diminished; and drain the spa completely every three months. Our spa has a cover to keep leaves and debris out, and we use a product to protect the spa's exterior shell and keep it waterproof.

To keep our spa's water safe, we test the water twice a week and use three bromine tablets each week instead of chlorine because it is more stable and less irritating. If the spa has been used frequently, I occasionally have to add shock to clean the water, or water clarifier. We prefer to run the filter longer rather than add water clarifier, but sometimes — like after a large party — it is necessary to add clarifier.

We think our spa is one of the best purchases we have ever made. Once you have made the decision to buy a spa, make sure you use it and take time to enjoy the experience. Our advice to other spa owners is:

- Maintain your spa. If you take care of the chemicals and keep the spa well-maintained, it will be available when you need it and will not require costly repairs. Improperly maintained pH can damage the heating unit, and improperly maintained chlorine or bromine allows bacteria to grow, making the spa unusable or unpleasant. If you clean your filter regularly, you will not have to replace it as often. We have had our filter for more than five years, and we clean it every week.

- Learn to do the maintenance yourself. Pool and spa maintainers can charge $15 a week or more for less than five minutes of work.

- Purchase a quality spa. Check out the manufacturer's warranty. There should be a guarantee of at least five years on the motor, and some places offer lifetime warranties on the shell. While it is true the price is not necessarily an indicator of the quality, purchase a spa from a manufacturer that has a proven reputation for quality and support and has been in business for a while.

- Make a conscious decision about the type of heating. The most popular forms of heating are electric and gas. Electric heating maintains the spa temperature over long periods of time, and it is a better option if you are going to use the spa often and if you would like to use it immediately without having to wait for the water to heat up. Gas heating is less expensive and is a better option if you are going to use the spa infrequently. This kind of heating also takes longer to heat the water — it takes 15 to 20 minutes to heat our six- to eight-person spa.

- Make an informed decision on the size of the spa. A two-person spa is less expensive to operate, but it will limit the number of people that can enjoy your spa. While we normally use the spa with only two or three people, it has been nice to have the option of having six to eight people over for a spa party. It makes a great gathering place after a sporting event or just to get together.

One final personal note: Purchase the bells and whistles that are important to you. I prefer strong jets for water therapy and comfortable seats. Try to avoid the frills like pop-up televisions, because who needs to watch TV in the spa? I also advise avoiding fancy drink holders or even sound systems, because these are just more gadgets that have the potential to break.

Making the Decision

Now that some of the health benefits of using a hot tub or spa have been discussed, it is time for you to decide what you want the spa to do. Spas have many different types of jets, circulation systems, and functions. This section will explain some of the different features that have to do with therapies and also equipment that can come with a spa that may be hidden under the cabinet.

For the potential owner, price is most likely an important consideration. Spas generally have a pretty good markup on them, and at the retail level, making a deal is not out of line. The trick to buying a spa is to pay for the equipment and not pay extra for the name. Usually, a good name means a better piece of equipment, but many spas use the same pumps, spa packs, and equipment as others. Adding a couple more jets allows some manufacturers to increase the price, which may not justify the equipment added. Always compare the equipment and warranties that are being offered. Another important piece of information is to find out where the nearest repair person is for your spa.

When purchasing a spa, the main consideration is that you get what you want. You do not want to invest a large amount of money in something that does not do what you really want it to do. From my experience, I have seen spa owners have their new toy delivered and because it does not quite live up to their expectations and the newness wears off, the spa just sits and wastes electricity.

It is important for you to find a dealer that will actually let you try out the spa to see if it is what you want. If all you need is a little stress relief, then any spa will help, but if you have an injury or area of your body that could use some additional therapy, make sure the spa you pick has the capability to do the job.

The following chapters will show you some of the equipment and other options available to you, including exactly what you need for a good spa. One factor that you have to consider is where you will put the spa when you purchase one. Will it fit where you want it to go? Of course, the availability of electricity needed to power the spa is a major consideration as far as added expense. These are some things for you to consider.

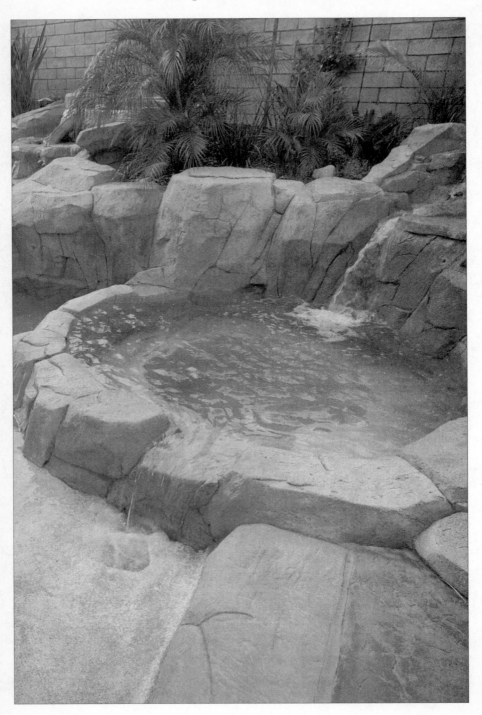

CHAPTER TWO

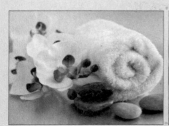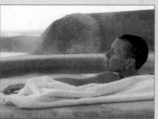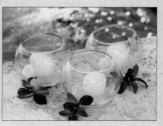

The Spa and Equipment

From this point on, all hot tubs and spas will be referred to as spas with differences pointed out as needed. All have one thing in common: the basic shell or container that holds the water. The volume of water that each can hold varies from spa to spa.

For the shell of a spa to hold water and the bathers in the spa, it must be made strong. Water weighs 8.33 pounds per gallon, or 2.2 pounds per liter. Say a spa seats four and holds 300 gallons of water. You are talking about 2,490 pounds of just water, not including the people sitting inside. Say the average person is 150 pounds. That adds another 600 pounds of weight. Now you are looking at more than 3,000 pounds that the shell must hold. When you include the weight of the initial spa itself, that lets you know that where you place your spa must be built to hold more than 2 tons of weight.

Your standard deck off your back porch may not support that amount of weight.

Soft-Sided Spas

There are many soft-sided spa manufacturers, such as Super Tub and Advantage Manufacturing. Some have external equipment, and some are built in. The important thing to remember here is that these spas have a surface made of vinyl and have to be carefully handled because the vinyl can be damaged easily. Chemical balance is very important in these spas because the sanitizers that are used can damage vinyl if not in correct balance. Even putting the chemicals in the tub can damage the spa if not done properly. The advantage to a soft-sided spa is when it is empty, one person can easily move it. They are good for the person who has a second home and just visits their property every once in a while. This is beneficial because the spa is not left with water in it.

Proper storage and cleaning is essential for the surface to last and not be damaged by residue left after draining the spa. While soft spas are usually the least expensive of all spas, one thing to consider is that you generally get what you pay for.

Acrylic Spas

A **spa shell**, or the exterior of the actual tub, usually starts out as a sheet of acrylic that sits on a mold. A vacuum is used to remove all of the air between the mold and the acrylic and helps form the shell to fit the mold properly. Once the shell is molded, either fiberglass and resins or acrylonitrile butadiene styrene (ABS) plastic is used to coat the outside of the shell to give it strength. Some manufacturers use spray-on foam to help strengthen the shell and advertise it as additional insulation.

The spa business is constantly changing, and other products are constantly being tried. One of the problems with this is it takes time to test for durability. The trick is to buy from a company that has been around for a few years and appears to be financially stable enough to continue to stay in business. It does no good to get a lifetime warranty on something if the company is not around to live up to that warranty. Also, it is important to note that usually a lifetime warranty means seven years, according to different state laws.

One advantage to acrylic products is they resist the effects of improper water chemistry. The chemicals used to maintain water balance can damage a spa surface if not introduced properly. A warranty on a shell should cover not only the structural part of the shell, but it should also have a surface warranty that covers **delaminating**. This is where the acrylic and backing — usually fiberglass or ABS — separates and bubbles appear on the surface. This warranty is especially important so the service department of your spa manufacturer cannot say it was chemical imbalance and not a manufacturing flaw. Replacing a shell is very costly and labor-intensive, and sometimes the entire spa has to be replaced due to this expense. To form a spa shell, a sheet of acrylic is heated, and then a vacuum is applied to suck the acrylic to the shape of the mold.

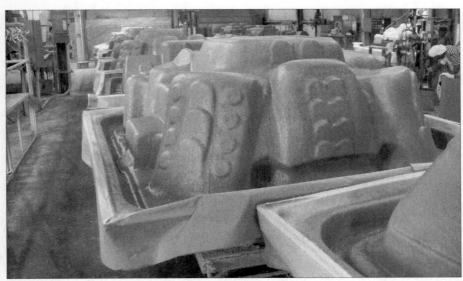

Figure 2-1 is a spa shell out of the mold. Courtesy of Premium Leisure

Cleaning

Use only the proper cleaning products that your spa's manufacturer recommends. Some household products are too harsh and can damage the surface, which will not be covered under a surface warranty. Some technicians recommend waxing the inside of the shell for added protection. However, be aware that the wax can dissolve under the heat and chemicals and subsequently may clog lines and filters over time. This also makes the inside of the spa so slick that it magnifies the chance of slipping, which may result in injury. This is one safety reason that it is recommended that you do not use the spa alone, or at least have someone supervise you while you are enjoying your spa in case you slip and hit your head or injure yourself in another way.

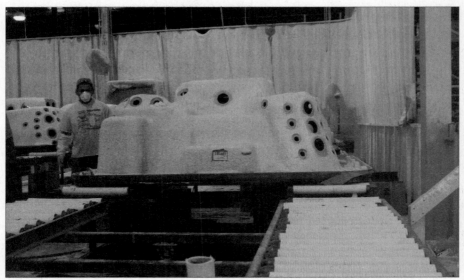

Figure 2-2 shows a shell with a layer of fiberglass rolled on the outside for increased strength.
Courtesy of Premium Leisure

Cabinets

The **spa cabinet** refers to the outer walls or skirting of the hot tub; this is used to enclose the spa's plumbing as well as for decoration. Up until recently, all spa cabinets were made of wood. The downside of this was that weather and humidity — not to mention the chemicals that are in the water that splashes over the side onto the cabinet — are harmful to wood. Some types of wood are resistant to the elements but not totally protected. Most people do not do any maintenance on these cabinets to help protect them so they last. A wooden cabinet may give you the look that you want, but it will not last forever. If you decide to use wooden cabinets on your spa, there are several types of wood from which you can choose.

Cedar cabinets cost a little more than pine and, if properly maintained, can generally keep their appearance. Redwood cabinets are more durable than cedar and require less work than other wood types — including cedar — but they also need some attention from time to time.

Mahogany cabinets are more attractive than the expensive oak cabinets that some manufacturers use. Both the mahogany and oak spa cabinets require much more maintenance to keep their appearance and protect the wood. Just like a pool, a spa's purpose is to use and enjoy, not to constantly work on. At this time, some of the alternative cabinets cost a bit more than some of the cheaper woods, but it is well worth the money.

All wood cabinets will require, at some time, some sanding and staining. The wood can absorb different things such as tannins, bacteria, mold, mildew, and different insect larvae. **Tannins**, which are polyphenols that destroy proteins and turn the wood dark, are stains from plants. Citric acid or chlorine can remove the stains so that the wood will look even.

If you enjoy finishing wood, you will have no problem with the maintenance required for a wooden spa cabinet. The cost to hire someone to refinish cabinets is expensive, but some people do not mind because they prefer the appearance of real wood and do not mind forking over the money to keep their spas looking great.

The alternative cabinets are made from different materials. Some are composed of polymer plastics and different synthetics. Polystyrene-based synthetic woods are a fairly new material; some have attractive patterns and some resemble wood. They do not last forever, though, and some can fade from the sun. It is important for you to check the warranty on your cabinet, but the new products for spas are getting better all of the time.

A good thing to look for when purchasing a spa is if the panels can be removed. Panel removal is important so the equipment and plumbing can be serviced. The less expensive spas will not have removable panels except for an access panel for the **ground fault interrupter (GFI)** or drain fitting. (A ground fault interpreter is a device that is designed to interrupt the electrical flow to aid in the prevention of electrocution.) *More about GFIs will be explained later in this chapter.*

If you have a wooden spa, it is important to remove the panels to treat the wood on the inside. Heat and humidity get trapped under the shell and can destroy the wood from the inside out. You will also want to check for leaks if you notice water around the spa.

One of the major structural parts of a spa is the frame that holds the outside of the cabinet, and this is what supports the shell and much of the weight. Some frames have solid bottoms made of wood, and some are not solid and the bottom of the spa is open with just the frame touching the ground. Using pressure-treated wood for the bottom and frame of your spa is a good place to start when choosing your spa. As most screws and nails rust, it is a good idea to see if stainless steel or other weather-resistant fasteners are used. The quality of a spa can be determined by what you cannot see as well as what you can see. When water is sitting on a concrete pad and a wood product is sitting on the concrete, a process called wicking may occur. **Wicking** is simply the wood absorbing the water from the bottom side and pulling it up into the wood, just like a wick in a hurricane lamp or the old kerosene lamps would do.

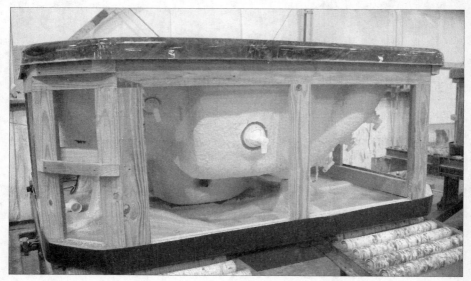

Figure 2-3 is a framed spa ready for plumbing and the installation of equipment.
Courtesy of Premium Leisure

Some of the better spa manufacturers like Premium Leisure use a **formed bottom**, which is a molded platform that the spa frame and cabinet sit on instead of wood or plywood. This acts as a protective barrier from the elements and provides a more solid frame for added strength. Such a bottom also lasts longer since it will eliminate wicking and is better able to withstand a damp atmosphere.

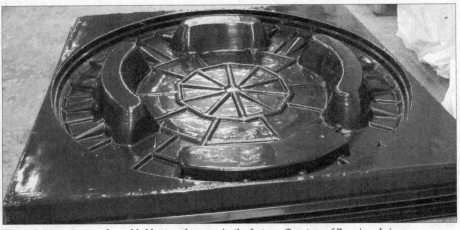

Figure 2-4 is a picture of a molded bottom for a spa in the factory. Courtesy of Premium Leisure

One of the most important things to remember about a spa is it is running off of electricity. Some of the less expensive ones run on 115 volts and cost more to operate, and the others run on 220 volts. No matter what voltage the spa runs on, a ground fault interpreter must be used. This is not the place to run your extension cord over to your spa and think you are safe. All electrical services for a spa need to be performed by a licensed and reputable electrician who knows how to wire a spa for service. Safety far exceeds the enjoyment that a spa delivers. Proper sizing of wiring and the use of the right GFI can save your life. Hardwiring a 220-volt spa is highly recommended — and is often required by law. **Hardwiring** is a permanent way of connecting a device by wiring it directly from the source of electricity to the subject without the use of plugs or connecters.

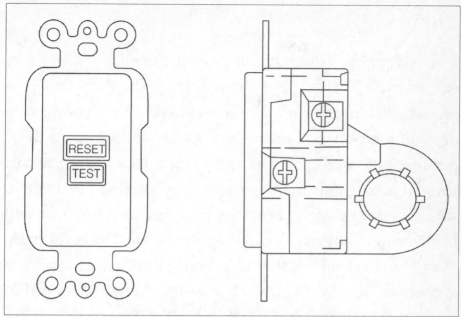

Figure 2-5 is a diagram of a common GFI breaker. Courtesy of Premium Leisure

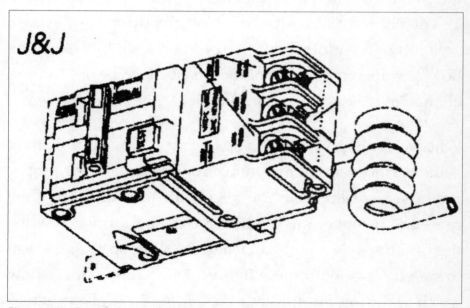

Figure 2-6 is a diagram of a common GFI breaker. Courtesy of Premium Leisure

Pumps

The spa pump is an integral part of the spa; this piece of equipment circulates the water through the filter and provides thrust for the spa jets. Some spas come with one pump or multiple pumps. You will hear of horsepower on these pumps, but horsepower is not what I look for on a spa. Instead of focusing on horsepower, pay attention to the flow rate of water that the pump can produce. The flow rate will be determined by the size of the jet the water flows through. Mini-jets need at least 9 to 12 gallons per minute to provide a good — but not painful — massage. Larger jets need at least 10 gallons per minute. If too large of a pump is used, the water will build up pressure as it flows through the jets. You do not want a spa that has so much power it will blow a hole through your kidney when you back up to the jet. The flow of water coming out of the jets needs to be only strong enough to massage in a comfortable — not painful — way.

When you are purchasing a spa, what you want to look at is the performance of the pump. You are looking for proper flow over horsepower. You also want to consider is flow rates and turnover rates, which are the performance statistics of the spa. It is a good idea to ask your spa salesperson to provide you with these figures. **Flow rate** is simply how much water moves through the piping in a given period of time, measured in gallons per minute (gpm). Flow rate needs to be calculated considering the piping and fittings the spa uses to get an accurate figure and not the maximum that the manufacturer of the pump claims the pump can deliver. **Turnover rate** is the amount of time it takes to circulate the volume of your pool or spa. Most states rule that a spa should turn over the total volume of water every 30 minutes.

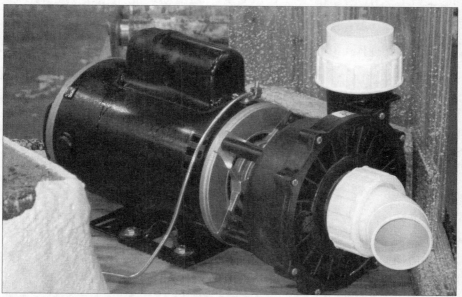

Figure 2-7 is a standard spa pump. Courtesy of Premium Leisure

Many different things in a system of spa plumbing affect flow rate. Every bend and turn of the plumbing adds resistance to the flow of water, and improper plumbing can cause a good pump to perform poorly. The real test to see if a spa flows well is to get in it. If a retailer is truly interested in selling you the product that they have and believe in that product, they will have a model that you can try out. If you

want to buy a new car, you surely take it for a test drive —
why should it be any different with a spa? If the salesperson
refuses to let you try out the equipment, then it is time to go
to the next store.

Multi-pump spas usually have a small circulation pump that
constantly circulates the water and keeps the temperature at
your pre-programmed level. Constantly running the water
allows it to circulate and be filtered; that is, if it is plumbed
that way. This smaller pump usually is less expensive to
operate than having the main pump kick on periodically to
bring the temperature back up to your preferred setting.

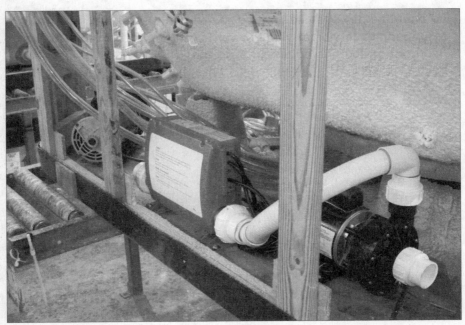

Figure 2-8 is a pump connected to the plumbing of a new spa. Courtesy of Premium Leisure

Unlike in a pool, the equipment concealed under the shell of a spa is not visible, so you have to either have the salesperson remove the panels for your inspection or believe what you are told. Always remember that salespeople usually work on commission, and some are like a good used car salesperson. Always refer to the manufacturer's data. When you go to the spa store and take note of the equipment listed, you can research the equipment on your own. For some people, a spa is fairly major investment, and you need to be sure that you get what you are promised as well as what you want.

Spa pumps usually do not have a trap with a basket on them because they are normally not exposed to the elements and are covered. A **trap** is part of a pump that has a lid and a basket to trap large debris before it enters the pump and filter. They are simple circulation pumps that are designed for easy removal if you can get to them. As with all equipment that is used in a spa, proper water balance is essential for the equipment to last.

When looking at the horsepower (hp) of a pump, you should understand what horsepower is. A 1 hp motor has a usable output equal to 746 watts of power. Watts are determined by multiplying the voltage by the amps. A 115-volt motor should draw 6.49 amps to produce 1 hp, or 746 watts of power. These ratings have to do with the efficiency of the motor. If a 1 hp motor draws more than the 6.49 amps, then it is not as efficient as a motor that draws the true 6.49 amps. This all has to do with the internal construction of the motor and wiring size.

Some of the newer motors are capable of actually producing more power than they are rated. This has to do with what is called a service factor. For example, say that you have a motor with a service factor of 1.25. The 1.25 rating is per horsepower, meaning the motor is capable of producing 1.25 hp even if it is rated as a 1 hp motor. The same is true if you have a service factor of 0.75. That rating means it is not as strong as a true 1 hp rating. That is why you will see some lower-rated impellors in some spa pumps. This rating and the differences in motors affect the flow rates.

A spa pump usually has a feature that most pools do not have. They have motors that can run on a choice of two speeds. This lower speed can be used for many different things. On spas that use the main circulation pump to maintain the temperature of the spa, the low speed is used to circulate the water while heating the water. If done right, water that is flowing slower through the heater will be heated faster while using less electricity. The common sales pitch is that it will result in less electricity used. However, this is not always true and the promise of less electrical use needs to be verified. Most of the newer pumps are more efficient and will use less electricity on low speed, but some will not.

Always ask for a specification sheet concerning equipment installed on your spa.

Skimmers

A **skimmer** performs the same function on a spa as it does on a pool — it skims the surface of the water for the debris that is floating on top of the water's surface. Many of the things that float on the surface of the water are undesirable (such as leaves and branches), and the skimmer removes them and moves them to the filter, where these items are contained in the filter media. These can come in many shapes and sizes. It is usually the choice of the manufacturer as to which type of skimmer to use; for quality spas, anything but a wall skimmer is appropriate.

Spa skimmers sometimes have a floating weir in combination with a basket and filter element under the cover, usually part of the basket. Some have a wall-mounted skimmer that is mounted in the side of the spa. The better spas have a **floating weir**, which is a cylinder-shaped device mounted inside the spa that floats at water level for better skimming; many also have separate filters for different pumps. Filters are of a certain cartridge type and can be cleaned.

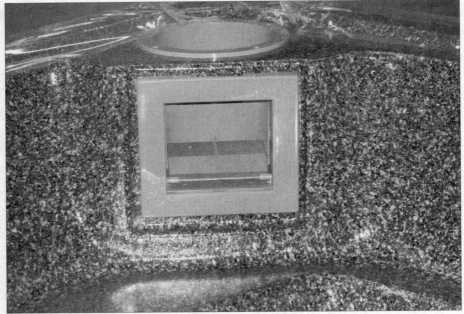

Figure 2-9 is a skimmer with a weir door. Courtesy of Premium Leisure

A strip skimmer is nothing more than a pipe mounted through the wall of the tub with an escutcheon, or cover. It has no basket, which means there is no way to clean the debris that enters the skimmer. Debris goes directly to the filtration system. Larger particles cannot be skimmed and just float in the tub until you physically remove them.

The skimmers that have baskets to hold the unwanted particles can either have a removable top on them for easy access or just have an opening on the waterside that allows you to take the basket out from the waterside. These usually allow debris to float out during removal and are easily spilled back into the spa.

A spa, however, differs from a pool in that a normal pool draws water from the intake, whether it draws water from the skimmer, main drains, or some other special suction line. From there, the water goes to the pump and through the filtration system before it returns to the pool. A spa, in comparison, draws water through the filters first and then to the pump. This is how the majority of the spas are plumbed and this is another reason why cleaning the filters on a spa is so important.

Filters

Spa filters take water from the surface of the spa to reduce impurities in the water, pump the clean water through the heater, and then return the water to the spa through the spa plumbing. The location of the spa filter varies, so check the owner's manual to help you find it. Most often, the filter is at least partially visible from inside the spa. The filter elements are cartridge-like in portable spas. On the permanent spas and pool/spa combinations, the filtration can be a cartridge, Diatomaceous Earth (DE), or sand filter. The type of filter used is, again, up to the manufacturer. However, the sand filter is almost outdated on residential pools because of the amount of water it takes to clean the filter. The cartridge filter is easier for most homeowners to understand and use, while the DE filter has the best ability to clean the water and remove debris but can be difficult for the average person to maintain properly.

The cartridge filter

A **cartridge filter** looks like an air filter out of a truck; it is tall, skinny, and round. It has pleats in the filter media that actually trap debris. The size of the filter and number of pleats determines the flow and filtration capability measured in square feet.

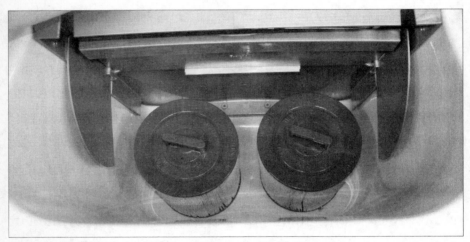

Figure 2-10 is a double-cartridge filter system. Courtesy of Premium Leisure

You can clean cartridge filters by spraying them with water to clean in between the pleats of the filter media. Body oils, lotions, and makeup can clog a filter, leading to the need for further cleaning. When the oils and makeup that float around the water attach to the filter, spraying the filter like normal will not remove them from the media. A simple way of cleaning is to put the filter in a bucket of water and add about a ½ cup of dishwashing liquid to a 5-gallon bucket of water. Let it soak for 48 hours, remove it, and spray off the filter thoroughly. You can also go to your local pool supply store and purchase enzymes used for filter cleaning. However, the dish detergent you use is much cheaper and will give you the same results. Dishwashing powder for your dishwasher will also do a good job.

Remember, it takes very little soap in a small container of water to produce suds, and you have to remove all the soap on your filter before you place your filter back into your spa. If you place a soapy filter into a spa, you will find your spa will start producing bubbles. A spa with even a small amount of soap on the filter will make many soap bubbles.

Another product that is reported to be very useful to clean cartridge filters is trisodium phosphate (TSP). You can most likely find this for less than $10. It can be used in conjunction with chlorine to help kill mildew and algae that could be trapped in the filter. However, it is worth noting that phosphates are algae fertilizers.

If your filters look like they are rusty, there may be iron present. To remove this iron, you can add citric acid to your filters. However, do not add citric acid to your spa to remove iron; you want to clean your filters in a bucket separately. If added to spa water, citric acid works so rapidly that you will have trouble flushing all the iron out of the water from the lines and equipment.

It is always a good idea to have a spare set of filters on hand for your spa so you can use one set of clean filters while the others are soaking and cleaning. Filtration is important to all spas to keep the water clean and remove undesirable elements from your water. Filtration is a very important element of proper, clean, and safe water. A clogged filter can limit flow to the pump and affects the performance of the water returning to the spa. This in turn limits the sanitation.

Many different manufacturers make replacement spa filter elements. Make sure that they can filter down to 20 microns or better. A **micron** is a measurement that equals 1 millionth of a meter. The higher the micron rating, the fewer particles it filters out, and the lower the micron rating, the better. A cheaper filter element that you choose with a larger micron rating will not perform as well as one with a better rating. Price sometimes pays for itself.

The sand filter

A **sand filter** is the least efficient of all the filters, as far as the ability to remove smaller particles. This type of filter uses graded layers of sand and gravel to remove debris from the water. The average particle size of a sand filter micron is 40.

Even though this is very small, it is not small enough to give you great service. The more debris that gets trapped into a sand filter, the better it filters. This type of filter also requires plenty of water to backwash it. **Backwashing** a sand filter reverses the flow of water so that the trapped debris will be forced out of the waste line and, if done right, leaves the sand clean to start the filtration process over again.

The Diatomaceous Earth (DE) filter

Diatomaceous Earth is a fine, soil-like material consisting of the ground fossils of diatoms; it is most often used as a filtering agent. The Diatomaceous Earth filter is by far the best filter on the market. Usually, they cost more than the sand or the cartridge filters, but the performance is great. They can filter between 3 to 7 microns on the average — these particles are so small you might have to pull out your microscope to see them. They also use a slide or multi-port valve. DE filters are not used on portable spas but are used on many permanent spas.

There are two main types of DE filters: a finger filter and a grid filter. The **finger filter** has long, narrow fingers that the water passes through. The newer, more efficient filter called a **vertical grid filter** is made of independent grids with a coating of special cloth. This is how a DE filter works: A coating of DE is usually poured into the skimmer, and it sucks up in the filter and coats the grids or fingers of the filter. Debris is caught in this media and gets trapped in the DE. When the pressure rises, just like with the other filters, you will back-wash the filter. The water passes through the valve and out the discharge port of the multi-port or slide valve. After the filter has been backwashed, you replace the proper amount of DE back in the filter.

If a **multi-port valve** is used, it usually has fewer positions than the sand filter. The basic functions of this kind of valve consist of the filtering and backwashing positions; the waste position, which allows the water to bypass the filter and go out the discharge port to waste; and the bypass or boost position, which allows the water to circulate but does not go through the filter. Whenever you change the position of a multi-port valve, you must turn off the pump first. Failure to do so can result in damage to the equipment and may even cause harm to you. The same procedure must be used if the filter is equipped with a slide valve.

A slide valve is a valve that usually has only two features: the filtration position and the backwash position. These types of valves are not optimal because you cannot drain water out of the pool without losing your DE.

The DE filter will clean a pool or spa faster and make the water clearer than the other two types of filters. DE filters do require periodic cleaning, but cleaning the grid filters is fairly simple. It is a good idea to schedule cleaning at the start of every season. Do not run the pool or spa without adding the proper amount of DE because failure to do this will clog the grids and can damage them. A properly maintained DE filter will work great for years.

Cleaning the grids in a DE filter can be done in three ways, depending on what has clogged them.

1. If you have treated for phosphates or have sand introduced in the grids — usually from the start-up of a new pool or permanent spa that was not cleaned properly before it was filled — then you may get away with separating the upper part of the filter and simply pressure-washing the grids with a hose to remove the debris.

2. If the filter is coated with lotions and oils, they may need to be soaked in a solution of soap that contains enzymes that eat the unwanted debris.

3. When a finger or grid is loaded with calcium or other metals, acid washing must be done to clean off the debris or you will have to replace the grids or fingers. Replacing these parts is expensive.

Suction Ports or Drains

Spa pumps do not suck water from a single place. They should have suction ports, sometimes called drains, which are usually mounted on the deepest end of the spa. These are designed to provide good circulation for all the water in the spa. Suction ports are not mounted on the floor so they are not stepped on.

These suction ports should be cleaned regularly to ensure proper flow of return water. A clogged screen can restrict the flow of water to the pump and limit the output flow into the spa shell. Not only does this affect the performance of the spa, but it also may damage the pump itself.

A permanent spa can have a suction port in the side of the bottom of the spa as well as a main drain. Due to safety regulations, a single main drain will either need a suction port that shares the suction in case of an accident or will have two main drains. This is to keep someone from getting trapped by the suction of the pump and causing injury or death.

Jets and Special Water Features

The **jet** — also referred to as a return jet or plain return — is the part of a spa that distinguishes it from a hot tub. The force of the water flowing from the pump through the jet opening pulls air through the hole to create the massaging effect spas are known for. There are so many different types of jets and jet features that the list is almost endless. A jet can just regulate water or mix air and water together. Some are adjustable and can change the flow of air that is mixed with the water to achieve a certain effect.

There are mini-jets that are smaller than the average jet, which generally has a ½-inch hole. There are rotating jets that swirl the water or pulsating jets that alternate flows of water and air to give you a massaging feeling. There are jets that move up and down and various ways to perform a task. Each spa manufacturer has a trademark jet or mixture of jets to provide a certain function. For example, Hot Spring® Spas has a jet that moves up and down and massages a person's spine. It all boils down to what you are looking for and the effect you want to get from a personal spa; for instance, whether the focus is on treating a particular part of the body or just for general relaxation.

Jets in modern spas are usually easy to change, should you want to purchase a different type of jet or need to replace a jet when one is damaged. *Most simply fit into a body fitting, which will be discussed in more detail in Chapter 3.* Some people may have different sets of jets to use, depending on what area of the body hurts and on what area they want therapy That is also a consideration when picking out your spa.

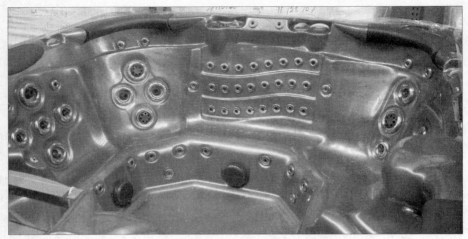

Figure 2-11 is a spa with three seating positions with different types of therapy jets. Courtesy of Premium Leisure

Whenever you have additional water features, more flow is required. Pick a spa that has the right equipment for you — this is where trying out the spa comes in — and not fancy features that have no therapeutic effect. If you have to supply water to features that are for looks, you will end up paying more for larger or better pumps and will also need more electricity to run those fancy functions. They are great for show but have no other purpose.

When it comes to non-water features, you also have an assortment of great choices. Some spas have stereo systems that use marine speakers (which have special enclosures for optimal use in water environments), CD players, or MP3 players, and some of the more expensive ones even come with flat-screen televisions. One problem with this type of entertainment built into a spa is that spa users will tend to spend excessive time in hot water, which can be dangerous. This is something that is important to consider when choosing a spa.

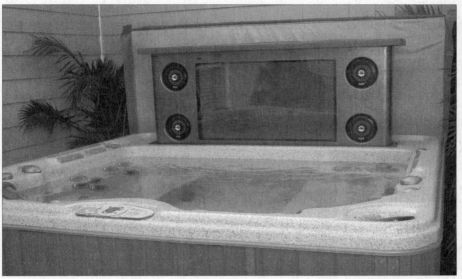

Figure 2-12 is an example of a spa with special non-water features; this specific spa includes a television. Courtesy of Premium Leisure

Covers

A **cover** will pay for itself over and over by retaining the heat of the water. Spa covers are insulated and designed to fit perfectly over the spa. However, not all covers are the same. Some are no more than solar covers, which hold in heat but will not support any weight, and then there are some that can hold plenty of weight; some can even hold the weight of a person walking on top. The heavy-duty covers are usually referred to as hard covers, while soft covers are usually thin bubble-like solar covers. When choosing a cover, remember that if a child or pet crawls on top of your spa and you only have a soft cover or solar blanket, they could drown in your spa. A cover not only saves you money, it can save a life.

Most removable covers have straps that can latch the cover in place. Unfortunately, most of the homeowners who have spas either have not installed these locking systems or do not use them. An accident can be fatal, so it is well worth your time to install and latch your spa when not in use.

Covers are like any other item you can get for your spa; there are many different types and they can offer different functions. The main thing is to get a cover that you can easily remove and install as well as one that provides protective security. Do not let price sway your decision in place of safety.

The American Society for Testing and Materials (ASTM) sets standards on spa covers based on many factors. One is how much weight the cover can hold and the other is perimeter deflection, which tests for whether the cover allows test objects (which are sized to simulate a child's head) to pass between the cover and the side of the spa, allowing the object access to the water. Tests also rate for surface draining, labeling, and securing or fastening the cover. An ASTM-rated cover is a good type of cover to have for your spa. The manufacturer or seller will always let you know when a cover is ASTM rated.

Covers are marketed based on the different types of materials they are made of and what kind of center core they have been manufactured with. There are also many different types of safety latches, many of which are just straps with plastic locks for security. A latch should not be easy to unlock for a child. Safety and security are the most important factors when deciding on a spa cover; after that comes the cover's ability to refrain from heat loss.

If you have children in the house, money should be no object in choosing a safe cover. The location of the spa should also be considered. A spa should always have a barrier or fence that prevents stray people and children from going for a dip in the hot water. Security, where a spa is concerned, is essential, and you can never be too safe.

Ozonators

Ozone is a highly reactive gas made of three oxygen atoms. The scientist Christian Friedrich Schönbein discovered ozone in 1839 when he smelled a unique odor during electrolysis and other electrical experiments. He recognized the odor as the one that occurs after a lightning strike. He named the substance "ozone" after the Greek word "ozein," which means, "to smell."

Ozone is "active oxygen" that contains three oxygen atoms per molecule. You can usually smell it after a rainfall. It occurs naturally in Earth's upper atmosphere from the sun's UV rays, and in the lower atmosphere during a lightning storm. The ozone layer protects us from harmful UV rays and is the center of controversy because it is being destroyed by manmade chemicals.

Ozone is used as a cleaner because it attacks impurities such as bacteria and viruses. The third oxygen atom, called a free radical, shatters carbon-chained molecules and breaks down harmful chemicals. The ozonator creates these molecules and mixes them with water through an injector in pools and spas to clean the water and fight bacteria. While some pool professionals feel that ozone equipment does not work because they cannot see it and readily test for it, the benefits of ozone have a long and detailed history.

In 1906, the city of Nice, France, was the first to build a water purification plant to use ozone. It has been used since the turn of the century to purify water and wastewater in municipal systems. In 1982, ozone was first used to purify bottled water. Ozone has been used for more than 60 years to purify pool and spa water. In the 1940s, ozone was used at the U.S. Naval Academy in Annapolis, Maryland, to clean its indoor pool. Since 1984, ozone has been used in all Olympic competition pools.

A major advantage of ozone is that it is very safe when used properly. It has no damaging effects on equipment. It leaves no chemical taste or smell and does not burn eyes or leave them red and irritated. It will not irritate or dry out skin, nose, or ears. It has no discoloring effects on clothing or hair. Most importantly, it is a strong oxidizer and it dissolves in water 13 times faster than oxygen. It is important for the spa because chlorine and bromine cannot kill certain organisms at the safe levels used in spa water. Ozone can kill E. coli and many viruses and does not dissipate in hot water. It is mostly invisible and is injected in the water by an ozone generator.

The technology behind ozone has developed greatly over the past few years. The United States is actually behind other countries in this technology. A company called Del Ozone in California has more than 1 million ozone systems installed worldwide and is going strong. Ozone is a product pool and spa owners should consider using, and one that a pool professional should recommend to customers who are having irritation problems with normal sanitizers. The majority of spa manufacturers build their spas with ozone systems installed or readily plumbed to add an ozone unit. Using an ozonator makes the water look crisp and clear.

Heaters

A typical spa heater may come in different styles but is generally either a stainless steel tube or a square box. Most on the inside look just like the elements that you will find in your hot water heater, but some elements are different. The highest cost of running your spa is heating the water and maintaining the water temperature, which is why a cover is so important, along with the safety aspect of the product.

A spa pack contains the guts of the spa and is what makes the spa work. The main components of the spa pack include the controller and the pump. Most spa packs have the heater included in the design of the pack. This is usually the one piece of equipment that always comes with the spa pack. The heaters that are located outside of the cabinet of the spa are different and are usually gas- or wood-powered heat.

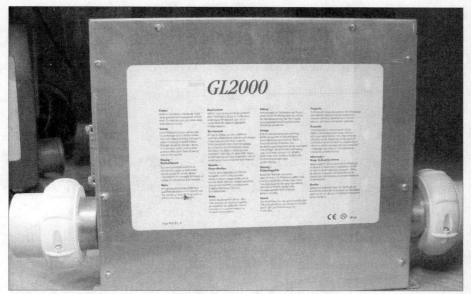

Figure 2-13 is a modern electric spa pack with the heater mounted through the bottom.
Courtesy of Premium Leisure

The heater in the spa pack has **limit switches**, which are sensors that determine the temperature of the water. By communicating with the controls electronically, the sensor shuts off the heat when it reaches the set temperature and turns the heat back on when the temperature of the water drops below the temperature programmed inside the controls of the pack. From a safety point of view, it is a good idea to have a thermometer for your spa to get an accurate reading of the spa water before you jump in. However, it is important to remember that these spa sensors do fail on occasion. When you are dealing with hot water, a few degrees difference in temperature can be very unpleasant and dangerous. Most spas now have thermal limit switches, which are designed to limit the temperature to between 102 and 104 degrees by turning off automatically when the temperature reaches that point. Do not tamper with thermostats or controls that have to do with temperature; they are put there with safety in mind.

On permanent spas, the heating system can vary greatly. You can use a heat pump, which draws the heat out of the atmosphere and transfers it to the water; a gas heater, whether natural or propane; a fuel oil heater, which are still in use in the Northern states; and a wood-fired heater. Depending on whether you are heating the spa continuously or just on occasion will determine the type of heating system you should use. Electric heating is the most expensive, followed by propane or natural gas heating. Wood heating is the most cost efficient because the source of the heat — wood — is inexpensive. Checking with your local pool and spa stores will help you make a decision, but also check more than one. It is a good idea to contact a pool and spa professional and get his or her opinion.

Gas heaters need to be turned on at least once every month for a few minutes to help keep the burner assemblies clean. Different insects get into the burner tubes of the heater and build nests that will disrupt the flow of gas and cause the flame to be less efficient. In some cases, this can clog up the heat exchanger with soot. This restricts the heated air, making the heater inefficient, and can damage components inside the heater. If the heater smokes excessively or makes a banging noise, you should turn it off and call a service professional.

A gas heater is a piece of equipment that should be repaired by a professional, not the owner. Propane gas is heavier than air, and it can "puddle" at the bottom of the heater. If you are messing with a gas heater and you have no idea on what you are doing, you can run the risk of seriously injuring yourself.

Permanent Spas

Certain companies make spa shells that are already plumbed and can be installed in a pre-built hole in the ground or another structure. These spas use equipment that is separate from the spa shell, located away from the spa instead of underneath, much like pool equipment; in fact, most of the equipment used for these kinds of spas — the pumps, heaters, and sanitation equipment — is the same that is normally used for pools. These spas can be very elaborate, depending on how much you want to spend, and they can perform various functions. The advantage of these spas is that you usually do not have to worry about cabinets, and the equipment is located away from the spa for easy inspection and maintenance. With these types of spas, usually gas heaters are the preferred choice over the electric heaters, and they are cheaper to operate than a portable spa. This is not always the case, though.

A basic pool/spa combination is usually just a circulation of water and maybe a blower (defined in the next section). There are some therapeutic advantages to these pool/spa combinations, but not as many advantages as a spa that has been designed for the purpose of therapy. The advantages are they utilize the pool water when the spa function is not in use, and the maintenance and water chemistry is usually not separate from the pool. Even though the water has to be heated each time you use the spa, a good gas heater can heat a 500-gallon spa very rapidly depending on the ambient temperature and the temperature of the water. These spas eliminate the chemistry needed for a separate spa and may have the ability to use a good filtration system to filter the water going into the pool and the spa. Because the spa is used for a short time and then the pool mode is put back on, the chlorine breakdown that typically occurs over 85°F is not an issue. (Chlorine starts to break down at 85°F, which is why many spas use bromine because it can withstand higher temperatures.) The water just circulates back to the pool, where the temperature is lower and the sanitizer can perform its duties. By overflowing the water from the spa to the pool and returning filtered pool water into the spa, it lowers the maintenance needed for a spa.

On the majority of the newer pools with spas, sanitation comes from a chlorine generator, or what is simply called a salt pool. This mild saline solution, when used in a spa, is healthier than some chemicals and also leaves the bather with a good feeling on his or her skin. The difference in bathing in a salt pool versus the conventional chlorine pool is very noticeable. The best way to explain it is to say it just feels better on your skin. The saline or salt water that is in the pool makes your skin feel softer and does not leave your skin feeling like it does after you have been in a chlorine pool.

Blowers

A **blower** on a portable spa only has one function, which is to blow air through holes in the seat and/or floor. It is not connected to the circulation system in any way. This is a controversial piece of equipment because some feel that even with the electrical protection involved, it is still unsafe. On a pool, the blower is mounted about 2 to 3 feet above the water line. However, on a spa, it is usually underneath the water line, which can lead to a problem if a check valve fails and water gets into the blower.

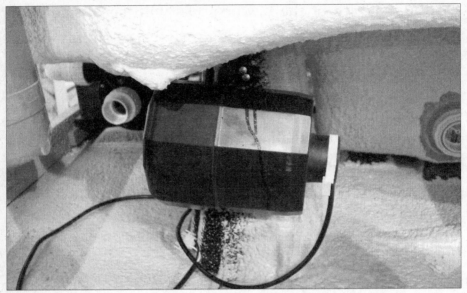

Figure 2-14 is a newer model of a spa blower mounted to a spa frame. Courtesy of Premium Leisure

A **check valve** is a device that is installed inline with the plumbing and allows water to flow only one way. If the check valve located at the blower on the spa is not sealing properly, water will flow into the blower, which should activate the GFI. This will break the electrical current going to the spa to protect spa users. This is another important reason to make sure an experienced electrician properly sets up your electrical connection to the spa. This can be an aggravating situation that makes you hate your spa, but not properly installing your electrical equipment also is dangerous.

A blower forces air either into a dedicated area of the spa to make the water perform in a rapid motion, or through the jets mixed with water to increase the activity of the water flow, making the jet more therapeutic. They are very useful, and if a manufacturer does not use them and has no confidence in their ability to make them work properly, then you should be concerned about the rest of the spa. A good check valve or two can cure any problem with blowers, and some have holes in the line of the blower to release any water that passes by the check valves.

Spa Packs

The spa pack is the heart of the spa. It usually contains the heater and the controls for the different functions of the spa. The control box in the spa pack will include not only the heater, but may have a built-in GFI, control circuits for the blower, an ozonator, different pumps, the lighting system, and any other additional equipment that is included in the spa. The spa pack is the unit that the spa-side controls connect to. There may be air-activated switches or electronic controls that have many different functions such as controlling the speed of the motor, lighting, and heating, and some controls regulate sanitizers.

Many different companies make spa packs, and they can have very limited functions or be very sophisticated and include multi-function switches, warning lights, and diagnostic features. Some have gold contacts and electronic circuit boards.

The standard spa packs consist of relays that connect a circuit to flow electricity to a particular piece of equipment when activated. If you open the cover, you will find a maze of wires, relays, and things that will confuse the average person. The newer spas use electronic components, and the advantage to this type of spa pack is that if one relay is bad, it can be replaced separately. The disadvantage is that moisture and humidity corrode and damage electrical contacts. From a service point of view, there are many little things inside the 220-volt control box, and it is easy to get shocked or make a small mistake and cook a part if you touch the wrong thing.

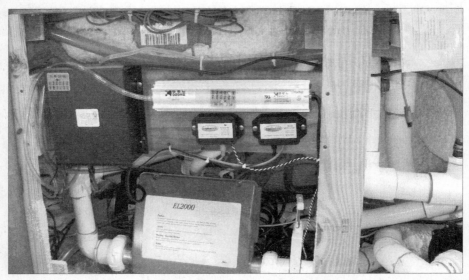

Figure 2-15 is a mounted spa pack (bottom center) with an ozonator installed above it. Courtesy of Premium Leisure

The electronic systems in the control box can perform many functions with a limited amount of space. They are very durable, and the moisture and humidity does not seem to affect them like you would think they would. Normally, the circuit boards are stepped down voltage, which means that the current runs through a transformer that lowers the voltage for the electronic circuit boards, usually to 24 volts. This makes it a little safer to service, but the disadvantage is when one thing goes wrong with a board, you have to replace the complete circuit board.

If you are not good with electronics, it is not a good idea to play with them. Even though most circuit boards are low voltage, there is usually high voltage running through them somewhere, and one mistake with a test probe or screwdriver can fry a board as well as yourself fairly easy. Just like a computer, static electricity can ruin a circuit board. The newer spa packs have what is called a **ground fault circuit interrupter (GFCI)** instead of the standard GFI. This unit not only protects the high voltage but also the low voltage on your control box. If your spa comes with an internal GFCI then you will not need to install a second GFCI externally.

As with all special equipment, make sure the electrician you use knows this type of equipment. If the electrician you hire is not familiar with spas, you could have a problem. Different areas have different electric codes, and some spas need to be bonded. **Bonding,** also called grounding, is additional protection for devices that work with water. It is a good question to ask your electrician if bonding is required in your area.

On the spas that I have run electricity to, I use an additional ground rod for additional grounding or a separate bond wire for the spa. It does not hurt to have additional protection. Let me give you an example: I have had this happen a few times, but recently I was at a pool and reached into the skimmer to remove the basket when I felt a slight shock. Because I was not sure if it was an electrical shock, I stuck my hand in there again and got the same result. I went to the controls and shut off the pump and the breakers that fed all of the pool equipment and still got shocked. This means that the pool equipment was not the reason for the shocks.

The owner had just built a new four-car garage and massive electrical conduit was installed on the side of the home with a new 200-amp service. I thought perhaps the ground wire might be touching either a hot line or the common line in something as simple as a light. Whatever it was, it was time to call an electrician. The owner acted as if it was our fault and nothing could be wrong with her electrical connections. So, we called our company electrician to go by and check the pool equipment, which checked out fine. When he opened the main service panel at the house that was just installed, he found the actual ground wire that connects to the rod that should be in the ground had been broken off.

To give you a little more information on pools and spas when in combination, there is a #8 AWG solid core copper wire that bonds everything together. The wire is attached to the rebar (a rod or bar used to reinforce concrete) in the pool shell, all equipment, the screen enclosure, the lights, and any other metal items that are around the pool and spa. The bonding wire connects everything, especially the electrical items, together to prevent electrolysis and is then grounded to the control box or a ground rod. Electrolysis is an electrical current that can cause a chemical reaction to occur and damages metals. In this situation, the entire electrical system of this home and garage was searching for a ground and with all these items at the pool being bonded together, it picked the bonding wire to use as a ground, which was why we were getting shocked. Once the ground wire was reattached to the ground rod, our problems went away.

Now, even when a good residential electrician installed the electric lines to the new structure, something can always go wrong. Do not gamble with the lives of your family and friends by cutting corners on the service to your spa. It is just not worth it.

For those who like to tinker — do not do it. Spa GFCI breakers usually are 60 amps, some 80 amps, and it only takes 1 amp to do you in. It you are not familiar with electronics or educated in electricity, then please call someone who is. Not only is it a safety issue, but you can also damage some expensive parts. The damage that can be caused by tinkering can cost you a new spa pack. Sometimes the whole unit is cheaper than some parts. Check with your factory for authorized service personnel.

Steps

When you are in water that is heated to 104°F, stay in for about 20 minutes and then decide it is time to get out of the spa, you may find that your body will not work properly. After being in such hot water for an extended period of time, you may find that your legs and other parts of your body will not respond the way you want them to. Being a little wobbly could be dangerous, and it is easy to fall if you have to reach a long way with your legs and you have limited strength. A good set of steps will help you get in and out of a spa easily and help prevent accidents. This is another reason to not use a spa by yourself or at least have another person in the immediate area in case you need help.

When purchasing a set of stairs for your spa, you want to pick out good, quality steps that support more weight than you think you will use. Some of these steps incorporate storage for your spa and have a very nice look to them. The other thing to look at when picking out steps is if they have a non-slip surface. The standard plastic steps can be very slick when they get wet, making them dangerous.

Pool/spa combinations sometimes are not built with the user in mind. Many of the spas are quite high off the ground and are difficult to get in and out of. The deck surfaces that use slick stone and tile make it very dangerous for a user once they get wet. Getting out of the spa and hitting your head on the edge is a very good possibility; hitting the deck surface and possibly breaking bones is also a real scenario. For those of you who have this type of spa, get a rubber mat and lay it on the deck beside your spa where you get in and out of the spa. This will eliminate the chances of your feet slipping out from under you.

Now that we have covered all the essential components of your spa and how they work, we will discuss the different aspects of a spa's plumbing.

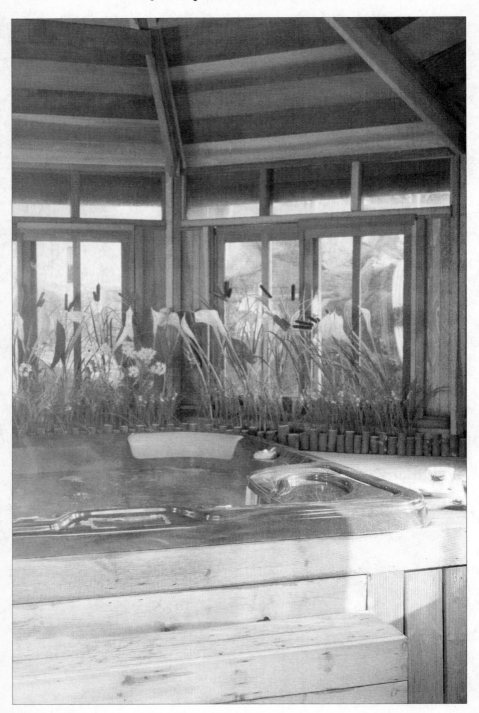

CHAPTER THREE

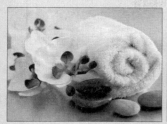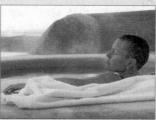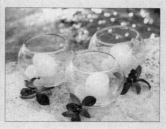

Spa Plumbing

The performance of a personal spa depends greatly on how it is plumbed. It can have good pumps and filtration, but if it is plumbed incorrectly, that can drastically change its performance. If the size of piping in the spa is too small, this limits the water's ability to flow properly. If it has too many turns, elbows, and couplings, then it has restrictions. Anything that changes the straight direct flow of water adds resistance and therefore limits flow.

When you look at your spa or the one on the showroom floor and you see that it is of considerable size, when it is full of water, the term "portable" seems like a joke. However, the word **portable** means that the equipment and plumbing does not extend outside of the spa but instead is all one unit. Another reason to call it portable is that if it were considered a permanent fixture, most municipalities would tax you on it.

It is important for you to know how things work and affect a spa, but the calculations can be difficult to understand because no company plumbs all the same. The best way to explain this is to start from the beginning. When you have a full container of water and it is free of air locks (bubbles or pockets of air that prevent the normal flow of water), the water flows from the skimmers and the main suction ports to the intake of the pump. As water flows through the pump, it creates a vacuum, which sucks more water. After going through the pump, the water leaves with a good flow and pressure — these work together. It takes pressure to create flow, but too much pressure will make the flow of water uncomfortable. Flow is what you really want, not high pressure.

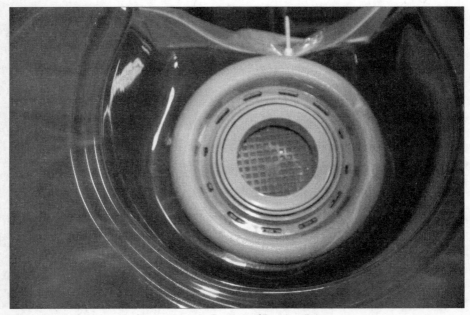

Figure 3-1 is a floating weir skimmer in a spa. Courtesy of Premium Leisure

Before the water reaches the pump, it usually goes through

a filter of some kind to keep the debris out of the pump. If you have a standard spa, it can simply go around the spa into the body that holds the jets. The normal body that the jets fit into usually has two separate connections, one for water and the other for air.

If you have multiple nozzles or jets, the line can run to what is called a manifold. This **manifold** is usually the same size as the internal dimension of the water line or larger. It has multiple connections for the water lines to go to different jets or sets of jets. The sizes of these manifolds affect the flow greatly because as water goes into the manifold, its natural flow is interrupted. When the water has to change directions, the water flow is restricted. If a manifold is sized wrong, what could be a nicely performing spa just turns into a water circulator.

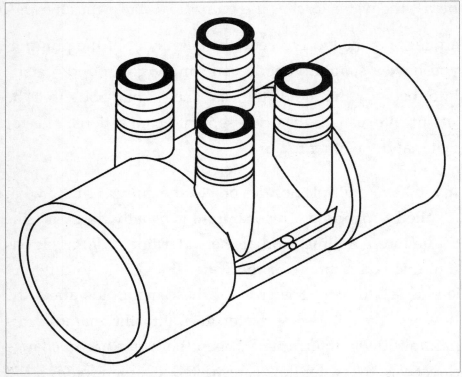

Figure 3-2 is a common manifold in a portable spa. Courtesy of Premium Leisure

When a spa is calculated for flow and performance, a great deal of mathematics goes into the design. The flow rate has to be correct for a certain set of jets to perform the way it was designed to perform. Simply put, if you added a couple more jets to your spa or a different massage unit, you could have to change the size of the pump. On a spa, this can create a flow problem by not providing enough water flow to function the way the jet was designed. It may not mean you need more horsepower, just a different pump that has more of a flow rate. Different size pumps with the same horse-power have different rates of flow.

Some spas come with standard massage jets, and some have added jets like mini-jets, flexible jets for the neck, or water fountains. Most of these not only have water flow valves but also what is called a **venturi valve** that allows for the air to mix with the return water in the jet itself before entering the spa. When air is mixed with water, it makes for a more powerful or turbulent effect. If the blower is plumbed into these, it can perform a very good massage. It almost makes the water blow out of the spa — and will do so if the spa is too full of water.

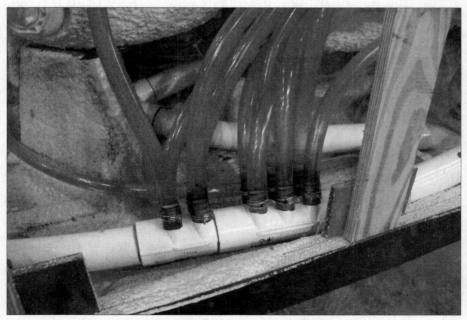

Figure 3-3 is a new spa with a plumbed pair of manifolds using clear, flexible tubing.
Courtesy of Premium Leisure

The air injection lines that mix with the jets usually have a regulator on them that allows a person to adjust the mixture of air and water to achieve his or her desired effect. Some jets do not have regulators because the jets themselves can sometimes be adjusted by the user by turning the outside face of the jet or by screwing the nozzle in and out. These adjustable nozzles can come in many different types and perform many different functions; some can rotate and are adjustable for flow and speed, and some can move up and down and in a circular motion. The search for the perfect spa jet is still continuing, which is why there are so many styles out there.

A spa that has no adjustable jets or regulators would be classified as a hot tub. It may circulate hot water, but the therapeutic effects are limited.

Spas with two pumps can have two suction drains, or they may have multiple skimmers with their own filters. The pumps can work together, or they may be set up to limit volume flow in one or the other. When two pumps use the same suction line, there is a strong possibility the pumps will fight for the water. If one of the pumps has a better performance than the other, the strongest one wins, which is why they are separated. This separation lets you have one part of the spa running during use, while the section you are not using does not run. Not only does this save electricity by only running the pump you are using, but it can also keep the water in your spa warm.

When a spa with venturi jets is running, the jets mix air. The air is the same ambient temperature that the spa is sitting in. If you are in a spa that is 102°F and the temperature around you is 70°F, then you are putting that air into the spa, which acts like a heat pump on the A/C mode. It will lower the temperature of the spa slowly by transferring the cooler air to the hot water. When you use a blower for a while, you can actually feel the temperature change unless you have a heated blower that heats the air before it is sent to the spa.

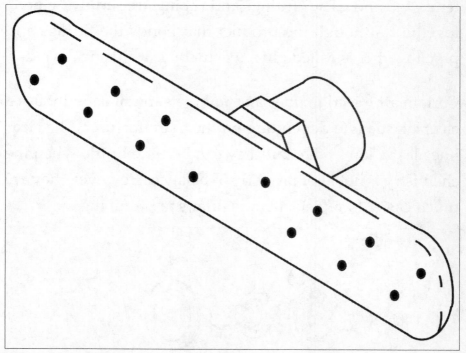

Figure 3-4 is an air injector mounted in a spa that mixes air with water without jet fittings.
Courtesy of Premium Leisure

Types of Products Used

The products used in spa plumbing are rigid poly vinyl chloride (PVC), chlorinated PVC (CPVC), flexible PVC pipe, and clear flexible tubing. Most fittings and parts that are used on a spa for water and air are made of these products. For the most part, they are lightweight, strong, and mostly chemical resistant. PVC fittings and parts are usually easy to make and are fairly inexpensive. The big advantage is that they are easy to use and easy to connect. The clear tubing is easy to replace and has a great advantage because you can see if you are having any scale buildup in your spa system. PVC and CPVC fittings and piping are simply "glued" together. Although the product that bonds the fittings and pipe together is called glue, it actually is a chemical weld.

Certain air injection lines and mini-jets might actually use a clear plastic line depending on the manufacturer. The clear lines last a long time, but they can become brittle when the chemistry is not kept properly in balance. However, they are much easier to replace than regular spa plumbing.

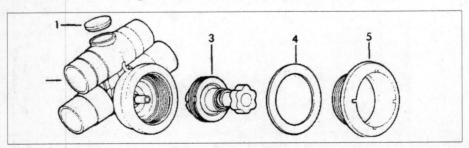

Figure 3-5 is a diagram of a jet body that incorporates air to be mixed with water.
Courtesy of Premium Leisure

This all goes back to trying the spa out. No matter how the plumbing is designed and installed, if it is done properly, you will feel the effect and get the desired action out of the spa.

On spas, like other things, sometimes the truth hurts more than it helps. For a salesperson to be successful, he or she used to have to believe in the product they were selling; however, now the sales industry relies on whatever someone can convince you to buy. A good salesperson is one who will actually provide you with the manufacturer's information before you ask for it. If they cannot back up the claims by written manufacturer's literature, then really get worried.

Fittings are connectors for spa piping, whether it is rigid or flexible. The different types of fittings used in a spa can be endless. Each manufacturer builds their own spa to their own design. Most manufacturers will constantly improve their spa's performance. Some do not improve their spas for cost reasons while others do not do it because they do not know better.

The trick to plumbing a spa is to prevent leaks. The housing that the jets screw into, usually the body of the spa, is installed into the shell. Normally, plenty of silicone is used to aid in the installation and to keep the housings leak-free. However, silicone can deteriorate with time when using harsh chemicals. Vibration caused from the water traveling in the lines and equipment can also cause leaks from time to time. This is why you need to periodically inspect the entire spa.

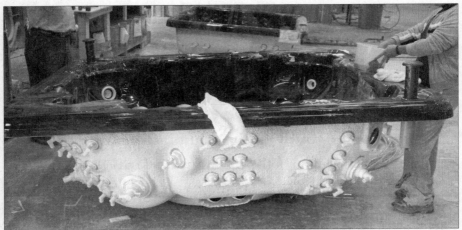

Figure 3-6 is a premium spa with the fittings and nozzles installed, ready for plumbing and to be put in the frame. Courtesy of Premium Leisure

Now that we have covered the plumbing systems you will need to be familiar with to maintain your spa, it is time to pay special attention to the water that will be in your spa. This next chapter will help explain everything you need to know about the water contained in your spa.

CHAPTER FOUR

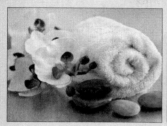 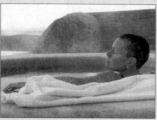 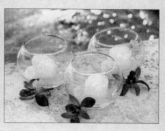

Water Chemistry

W ater chemistry is the most important concept to understand when you own a spa. Some consider a spa to be just a small pool, and that may be true in some respects, but when it comes to the managing proper water balance, imbalanced water can be unpleasant and even dangerous. What you are dealing with in a portable spa is a volume of water usually less than 500 gallons because the average portable spa holds between 200 to 400 gallons of water.

As temperature rises in water, the bacteria thrive. What is more important to consider is that viruses and fungi also like the heat. The steam that rises off the water contains spores of fecal matter, skin, and anything else that comes off a bather. This is a problem with public spas. Being in an indoor spa creates additional problems because without the fresh airflow, these spores cannot be blown away and are breathed in by bathers.

When the jets of a hot tub or spa are turned off, bacteria, scum, and fungi that are left in the piping or the filters come into the water in great quantities. When you turn the spa on, you get a large amount of this unwanted debris rushing out of the pipes, and what does not enter your body through your pores enters through your lungs. Hot water opens the pores of your skin and allows the foreign matter to enter your body. When the jets of a hot tub or spa are running, they create a mist, which is what enters your lungs.

This is all intended to make you aware of what can happen if improper maintenance and chemistry of hot water is not followed. Maintaining the sanitation in a spa and a good cleaning from time to time will keep you from having problems.

The guidelines that are set by the different water maintenance agencies are designed for the concern of the safety for people using a spa. Too many people think the art of balancing a spa is something they do not need to pay much attention to, but whenever the health and well-being of the human body is concerned, you should take it very seriously. Particular attention should be paid to adding chemicals to water. Never add a chemical to your spa that you just want to try or because you ran out of options. Problems that can occur with the misuse of spa chemicals can turn deadly.

What Water Wants, It Usually Gets

If the water needs something, it will attempt to take it from whatever is available. If it needs a little calcium, it might attempt to take it from the surface of a pool or spa by pitting or etching the surface. If it needs to get rid of something like scale (a thin film or incrustation of oxide), it has no problem depositing it wherever it can. This is called balance. You have to balance the water to give the water what it needs to keep it from doing damage; you should also balance the water to protect the pool and the equipment. You want to keep the water in good balance or else the water will take over and do whatever it wants to.

Almost every chemical you add to your spa can and will have an effect on some other aspect of the balance of water. If all water were almost perfect, balancing would be no problem. However, there are many things in water that could affect the chemistry. Whenever you add a chemical to adjust one thing, you can be sure that it has an effect on another. Balancing is an art and a science.

Dealing with water chemistry involves the important aspect of chemical safety. The first rule of chemical safety is that you never mix any chemicals. Your basic pool and spa chemicals mixed incorrectly could make a chemical explosion, and can also produce gases that are fatal. It is important when you store chemicals at home to keep them protected and away from the general public, especially children.

Rule No. 2 is always pour acid into water and never water into acid. This mainly applies to liquid muriatic acid. Dry acid can be added to the spa directly or it can be pre-dissolved. Care should be used with acid as it is corrosive and the body does not like acid. If acid gets on your clothing or body, rinse the area thoroughly with water. Sometimes the acid we use in spas, especially the liquid kind, will get on you, and it takes a few seconds or even minutes for you to discover that your skin is burning. Usually by that time, some damage has been done, and acid burns take time to heal and are also very painful. Aloe vera works very well on acid burns. If you spill muriatic acid on yourself and rinsing it with water does not seem to help, then you can put baking soda on the area and it will render the acid to neutral.

Rule No. 3 is if stored chemicals are old and if the containers are rotting, discard them in the proper way, according to the manufacturer or local codes concerning hazardous chemicals. Different municipalities have different rules on disposal of chemicals. If chemicals are in containers that are not properly marked, discard them.

This may not mean a lot to you now, but managing this small amount of water requires patience and carefulness. There are many technical definitions of balanced water, but this term simply means that all the chemical parameters are where they should be. Sanitizers are not a part of balanced water but do change some of the other parameters when introduced to the water. If using the Langelier Index of water, the balance is zero.

The **Langelier Index** is the measurement of saturation of your water. In the 1930s, professor Wilfred Langelier was hired to figure out how to create a thin layer of scale on pipes that carried the water supply for a city water system. The reasoning behind creating this scale on pipes was that if a thin layer of scale lined the cast iron pipes, corrosion would be limited. Later on, this would be adapted for the pool and spa industry to determine balanced water. The index is rather complicated, but it is an accurate measurement of balanced water.

There are four major factors that are considered for balanced water that affect the index of saturation. They are pH, total alkalinity, calcium hardness, and temperature of the water. As previously stated, balanced water has a saturation index of 0. If the saturation index is plus or minus 0.5 pH, the water is considered balanced. If the readings are lower than negative 0.5, it is considered corrosive. If it is greater than positive 0.5, it is considered to be scaling.

Some good pool shops that test water use the Langelier Index, but there is the problem with that. The water that you take out of your spa at 102°F will not be that temperature by the time you bring it to the pool shop. Therefore, the test will not be totally accurate. If you take your pool water in and it sits in your hot car for a period of time, then the opposite occurs. Some test kits, such as the Taylor kits, have a water balance calculator that helps you determine the saturation index of the water. This would make it possible for you to adjust your spa at home correctly. This is also the manufacturers' recommended way to adjust your water.

Balanced water is non-corrosive and non-irritating. Water that is out of balance can damage equipment and your spa, and it will irritate the skin and eyes of bathers. When water is corrosive, it can become very aggressive and can even dissolve concrete and metals. Spa water that is out of balance can eat the metal inside the heat exchanger of a heater, creating a very expensive repair and dissolving the heating element of the electric heater used in spas. This makes for a very unhappy spa owner.

In this book you will read about sanitizers and oxidizers. A **sanitizer** is a chemical agent used to oxidize bacteria, and an **oxidizer** is a chemical that releases chlorine, bromine, peroxides, and persulfates, or any other chemical in the halogen family of chemicals used to treat water. An oxidizer kills or inactivates a microorganism in the water of a spa. When sanitizing, the oxidation process takes effect. As defined by Taylor Technologies Inc., **oxidation** is when organic contaminants that a bather and the environment introduce — hair spray, deodorant, suntan lotion, body oils, or perspiration, for example — are burned.

Because a spa has a smaller volume of water, things tend to make a greater difference than if it were a 15,000-gallon pool. The owners of pools take for granted many things compared to spa owners because a pool with a large volume of water dilutes more things that could possibly be dangerous to their health. For that reason, pool owners tend to not pay attention to things they are not used to dealing with.

Here are some examples of problems that can occur in a spa. There was a particular spa that was located indoors with limited ventilation, even though it is not recommended to have a spa in an area of poor ventilation. However, in1999 in the Netherlands, a hot tub on display at a flower show contained Legionella, which is a version of Severe Acute Respiratory Syndrome (SARS.) Legionella can lead to pneumonia. This disease made more than 200 people ill and 32 died. A public bath in Japan was the source of 34 infections of Legionnaires' disease, and three people died.

A more recent illness known as the hot tub lung disease is associated with Mycobacterium avium complex (MAC). This disease is caused when you breathe in tiny biofilm particles in the mist of a spa, and some of the conditions include pneumonia and hypersensitivity reactions.

Chlorine is not effective enough in hot water to kill these unwanted creatures because its effectiveness is limited at temperatures warmer than 85°F. An alternative sanitizer is recommended. Bromine would be a good sanitizer with the addition of ozone. These chemicals will be discussed further in Chapter 5.

Very potent bacteria called Pseudomanas aerginosa will thrive at water temperatures around 104°F, so it is good to include a solution that will kill bacteria at high temperatures. As you probably know, fecal matter — which, unfortunately, may end up in your spa — can carry E. coli. When water is heated, the chance for the growth of bacteria and other things occur more rapidly than if the bacteria were in cool water. If a spa is not maintained properly, it could be hazardous to your health. That is why if you are not going to maintain the spa properly and safely, do not get one, or hire a professional to do this for you. A proper ozonator kills E. coli and other bacteria.

Pool and spa technicians introduce poisons into the same water that you are in. There are very few things used in water chemistry that are not poisonous; however, these potentially toxic substances are diluted to safe levels. Not only does water affect your body when the chemistry is out of whack, but it can also eat away the metals in your equipment. If it can dissolve metals, consider the effect it is having on your body.

The advantages to this book are that you can keep referring to it for reference when you forget how to do something. There is a great deal of information you must learn to properly maintain your water, but it is not difficult. When you get the basic understanding of water maintenance, it will become fairly easy for you.

Certain things affect water, and these must be controlled in prescribed levels, usually measured in parts per million (ppm). Sanitizer levels, alkalinity, calcium hardness, stabilizer or conditioner, and total dissolved solids (TDS) levels are all measured in parts per million, whereas pH is measured on the pH scale. All of these measurements will be important in determining the balance of your water and will be important when you start conducting water analysis.

Basic Water Analysis

Water testing is a simple procedure that the spa owner needs to perform on his or her spa at regular intervals. The advantage to a spa over a pool is that with the smaller amount of water and the amount of water circulation, you can dissolve and circulate chemicals faster and retest them in a matter of minutes. Every week — if not sooner, depending on use and bather load — is recommended for water testing.

To get a sample of water to test, you may want to use a laboratory wash bottle, which is a type of bottle that can be purchased from a chemical supplier; when you fill it and put the lid back on, it has a straw-like pipe that sticks out of the lid. When you squeeze the bottle, a controlled amount of water comes out, and you can accurately put the proper level of water in each test vial, which is extremely important because the wrong water level in the test vial will create incorrect readings. Also, most bottles of reagents work more accurately if you hold the bottle straight up and down instead of at an angle. You can then take the water sample away from a spa return and try to get the sample approximately 12 inches below the water line. Being near a return jet can give you false levels because the sanitizer equipment is the last place water passes through before it enters the pool; therefore, the concentration of chemicals will be strongest near a jet, so it is best to test away from these. It is best if the spa has circulated for a few minutes before the sample is taken so you can get an accurate reading. Always test your water before adding any chemicals.

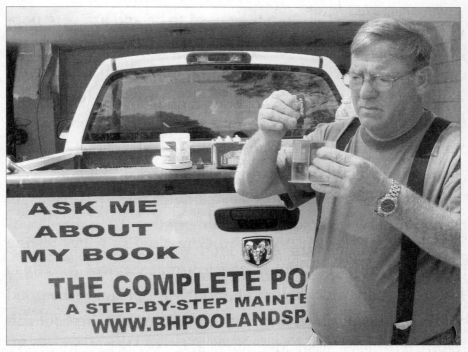

Figure 4-1 is the "Pool Doctor" Dan Hardy testing water and showing that the reagent bottles need to be straight in order to get an accurate drop for testing. Courtesy of Dan Hardy

Many different companies make test kits for spas. There are liquids, tablets, electronic measuring devices, and test strips. All of these methods, if used properly, can do a good job.

Liquid test kits are mostly Orthotolidine (OTO) and Diethyl-p-phenylenediamine (DPD). DPD test kits are preferred by many states, most likely because OTO is a very poisonous and hazardous chemical. Some states have even banned the use of OTO. Due to the danger of this chemical, make sure if you use an OTO test kit that you do not dump the tested water back into the spa or pool.

Test strips are better than they used to be and are very popular with the homeowner — and even some professionals because they are more convenient. These are like the litmus paper used to test urine or blood but instead designed to work on certain aspects of water chemistry. Care must be taken to follow the manufacturer's instructions because many test strips vary in the procedure used to get an accurate reading.

Electronic probes are also another method of water testing you can consider; these small electronic devices have also come a long way in a very short amount of time. The good probes are expensive, and they are not made to test for calcium hardness, total alkalinity, and cyanuric acid levels. There are testers made to measure salt, sanitizers, TDS, and pH. The salt tester is primarily used for the salt pools.

Liquid test kits generally work the best. High levels of different chemicals seem to affect the strips more than the liquid tests, and you can get interference fairly easy. **Interference** is when two elements do not work well together and provide false or difficult readings. Over time, you will be able to notice that interference is affecting a test.

Owners or hired professionals must test the spa water on the premises as soon as it is taken. You should not take spa water to the pool store because the temperature change your water will encounter as you take it to the store will affect the results of the test. It may not be a big difference but could be enough, with small water volumes, to cause you to make a mistake in proper chemical dosages. This is the accident you want to avoid.

Normally, a spa does not need any stabilizer because it is usually covered so the sun does not affect the sanitizer levels (sunlight depletes chlorine). Because it would be very easy to overdose your spa with stabilizer if you are using chlorine, do not use any stabilizer. Trichloro-s-triazinetrione, or trichlor, tablets already have stabilizer in them, and bromine does not use stabilizer.

The task of the professional or owner is a very simple one: Keep the water balanced to avoid any problems and unnecessary repairs. There are parameters that are set to determine the proper balance of the water. This section will go into testing sanitizer, pH, total alkalinity, and calcium hardness.

If you are having a particular problem with your spa and your neighbor or friend is having the same problem, while your problems may be similar, there may be different reasons why these problems are occurring. Each situation is unique and calls for different approaches.

Sanitizers are not part of the basic water balance. They do affect the testing, and each chemical has its own characteristics, some of which affect the others in many ways. This will be discussed in Chapter 5. Each sanitizer has a different pH level, which will affect the balance. However, the pH level is not the first thing you adjust; you always adjust the total alkalinity before the pH.

Total Alkalinity

Alkalinity can best be described as a "buffer." **Total alkalinity** (TA) is basically the measurement of the ability of your water to resist wild and sudden changes in pH. These sudden changes are called **spiking**.

Because every chemical you add to your pool has different pH factors, the total alkalinity is very important to keep sudden fluctuations down and decrease the chance of spiking. This is one of the main reasons that you always adjust your alkalinity before you adjust your pH. A high chlorine level will also throw your TA test off because chlorine has its own pH. The colors of the water in your test results will not be what you are used to, so you need a chlorine neutralizer.

Low alkalinity can result in corrosive water that can damage heaters. It can dissolve metals and stain walls. High alkalinity levels scale water, which can cloud your water and reduce circulation. Also, when your alkalinity levels are low, then **pH bounce** — the rapid spiking and fluctuations of pH — can occur. High alkalinity readings usually cause the pH to drift upward, but not always, depending on your sanitizer.

The recommended levels for alkalinity under the 2005 ANSI/NSPI Guidelines for chemical parameters is 60 to 180 (these recommended levels are not re-evaluated every year, so these are the most current figures at the time of publication).

Hydrogen Power (pH)

A standard that the beer industry started using back in the early 1900s was pH, which stood for "potens hydrogen," a Latin term meaning "hydrogen power." This is basically the measurement of acidity that is caused predominately by the hydrogen ion.

A pH scale runs from 0.0 to 14.0, with a pH reading of 7.0 considered neutral. If the water is under 7.0, it is considered acidic, and if higher than 7.0, the water is basic or alkaline. To give you an example, the pH scale is logarithmic, which means that every whole unit increase is 10 times its predecessor. What this means is that if you have a pH of 6.0, it is 10 times more acidic than a pH of 7.0, and a pH of 3.0 is 10,000 times more acidic than a pH of 7.0. That shows you how important it is to control the pH in a pool or a spa. The water is kept slightly alkaline, and the recommended parameters are for a range of 7.2 to 7.8, with the ideal at 7.4 to 7.6. If you have a low pH and chlorine is introduced into the water, it can be very corrosive. If a pool or spa is using bromine as a sanitizing agent, it is more critical. Bromine is very aggressive and can dissolve metals quickly. When you have a chlorine reading of 7.2, your chlorine works at 80 percent of the effectiveness of the product you are using. At 7.8, it works at 20 percent. Keeping your pH in the lower range can improve the effectiveness of the sanitizer, but you have to be aware that it is more corrosive if the levels get too low.

High pH makes chemicals come out of solution and turns those un-dissolved into solids. These solids are one reason why water is cloudy when it has a high pH reading. A high pH level makes chlorine less effective in preventing algae and bacteria growth, and it is also one of the major causes of skin irritation and itchy eyes in bathers.

You can lower the pH level with acid *(which comes in various forms that are discussed in Chapter 5)*, and, in some cases, you raise pH with soda ash, or sodium bicarbonate. It is important to remember never to mix any form of acid with any other chemical that you use, and always pour acid into water, not the other way around. Chemical reactions can and will occur if the absolute safety of these chemicals is not used. Always refer to the product safety labels and Material Safety Data Sheets (MSDS).

Once a chemical is added to adjust the pH factor of your water, it has to mix and stabilize before you can get an accurate reading. You should wait at least 15 minutes with all jets and the blower running before retesting your water, and then if it is questionable, give it another few minutes. This is all determined on how well the equipment was designed and if it is functioning properly. The turnover rate of a public spa is usually 30 minutes, which means that all the water will be circulated every half hour. You will want to restrict the use of the spa for an hour to allow for the chemicals to be dispersed so there are no problems. Safety is the key here.

Some problems that occur with low pH are dissolved metals, stained walls, and decreased sanitizer. In vinyl spas, the liner can wrinkle. Bathers may also experience skin and eye irritations. When the pH is high, the problems can be the scaling of lines and the surface as well as the internal components, which complicates things.

It is very possible to get a false reading or interference when testing pH. Usually, this is due to a high sanitizer level. Chlorine at 10 ppm and more can easily give you a false reading.

To eliminate something causing interference in your water, add a couple of drops of chlorine neutralizer, such as sodium thiosulfate. This will kill the chlorine, and your test should return to normal. If there is no change in the test after doing this, then look for something else out of whack or find out if something was added to your water. If you cannot figure it out, drain, clean, and refill your spa.

Repeat

When testing your water, if one level in your spa, such as your chlorine level, is extreme, then interference can give you a false reading. Bromine also has this capability. If interference is apparent because your test water is discolored, you can simply retest and add an additional drop or two of the first reagent, thiosulfate, which neutralizes chlorine. Never take a test reading after adding chemicals; always test the water first before any additions are made. The addition of other chemicals, which have their own characteristics, can give you the wrong readings.

Calcium Hardness

Hardness readings of pool and spa water are different than hardness readings for drinking water. Hardness readings focus on the calcium level in the water. The other element associated with hardness is magnesium, which is a concern in drinking water. Magnesium does not scale, so it is primarily left out of the pool and spa industry. If none or a small amount of these items are not present, that is considered soft water, which is not desirable for spa water. Many homes have water softeners that are not plumbed separately from the faucet used for the spa, so calcium chloride is added to put the levels at the proper recommended level. This is more critical in concrete spas than in acrylic spas. The manufacturers do recommend a certain calcium level for proper balance. Water will scale more when hot because calcium becomes hard to dissolve as temperature rises.

Another problem with soft water in a spa is simply the water is too pure. It needs some junk in it. For people who have water systems in their home, they know that it takes less soap to make good suds in soft water than it does in hard water. When you have pure water without many minerals, then very little un-rinsed soap from your clothing and some oils can make foaming more of a problem. It appears that the harder the water, the less of a problem you have with foam. Hardness levels can sometimes be misread when metal levels of over .03 ppm are present in the water. There are ways to correct the interference these elements cause, depending on which test kit you use.

Low calcium can cause your spa's plaster to dissolve, concrete to pit, your tile grout to dissolve, and some decks may even pit. High calcium can plug lines from scale buildup, which can result in poor circulation, cloud the water, and ruin a spa heater and a chlorine generator, if you have one.

Proper hardness levels the ANSI/NSPI recommends are 200 to 400 for pools and 150 to 250 for spas. A level of 250 for a concrete spa and 200 for an acrylic spa is recommended.

Unfortunately, when the calcium level gets too high, the only way to rectify it is to drain the spa. Draining a spa should be a regular function of the maintenance, and when this should occur depends on the bather load.

Temperature

Technically, temperature is not a property of chemicals. However, temperature is a major factor in determining how the chemicals in the water interact with each other. The temperature of your water affects total dissolved solids (TDS), pH, and the other factors in water maintenance. The warmer the water, the less soluble calcium carbonate is. The higher the temperature of water, the more gases that are released due to decreased solubility, and this release of gases leads to high pH. The quick and easy way to say this is that the gases are acidic, and when acid leaves the water naturally, the pH rises, making it more basic.

Cyanuric Acid (Stabilizer)

A stabilizer is not needed in a spa. The main point that needs to be made about cyanuric acid is that it is dangerous. Any acid, whether it is the acid from a soda pop or muriatic acid, will form a poisonous gas.

Total Dissolved Solids (TDS)

Another big difference between a pool and a spa is that when you are dealing with a large volume of water in a pool, it can dilute many things, and most can be filtered out. In a spa with a small volume of water, there is not enough water to have many things floating around in it. TDS, which is **total dissolved solids**, is defined as the measurement of everything that is dissolved in your water.

An easy way to describe TDS is like a glass of tea. You can add a teaspoon of sugar and it dissolves. If you add 3 teaspoons of sugar, this makes the TDS level high because the saturation level of the tea is so high that there is no more room to dissolve any more sugar. A level of 1,500 ppm of measured TDS is high in a pool or spa, and draining is required to remove this high level and replenish with clean water. A salt pool is the exception to this rule.

The other advantages of a spa with small volumes are that whenever the water becomes unmanageable or cloudy, you just simply drain and replace the water. This needs to be done on a regular basis. There is a basic mathematical solution that seems to work when you are trying to determine when to change the water in your spa. Say your spa holds 450 gallons of water. You take the volume of water and divide it by three, which is to 150 gallons. Now look at how many bathers you will have in your spa — say it is three. Divide the 150 gallons by three and you get 50. The general rule in this case would be to change your water every 50 days. So the equation for when to change the water is as follows:

(Water volume) ÷ 3 ÷ (number of bathers) = (how frequently to change your water)

Many other things affect that figure, however. To follow are some questions to ask yourself about the variables that may affect the TDS in your spa.

Do you shower before you enter your spa? Not showering can cause perspiration, body oils, fecal matter, and dirt and grime that have gotten on you during the day to dissolve in your clean water.

Do you remove your makeup before entering your spa? Not doing so will leave slime on the edge of the spa at the water line, and this will get lodged in your plumbing. It is hard to clean out of your piping. Lotions are also a no-no.

Do you use a laundry detergent that contains phosphates, or does your washer not take out all of the soap? Using the same swimwear and washing it every time is not good. Even a little soap that is left on your clothes can contaminate the water and will surely make a bubble bath. It is recommended that you rinse and take your swimwear off, then let it air dry or dry it in your dryer without using dryer sheets. It is best to go nude in a spa — that eliminates the problem of phosphates and soap. This may be impossible, however, if you have a family or have your spa in an area where others can see you.

Whenever you are in doubt or having problems with your water balancing or not clearing up, drain it. Do not waste money on various chemicals when water for a spa is cheap. For those who use a defoamer to remove the bubbles and soap foam, after three applications to kill the foam, it is time to drain your spa. Make sure you flush and clean the surface very well before filling. Because filtration is also an important component of a spa, make sure that regular maintenance is done on your filters. *This is explained in Chapter 12.*

Recommended Guidelines for Water Quality

The following are the recommended guidelines for spa chemistry from the National Swimming Pool Foundation in 2005.

Parameter	Minimum	Ideal	Maximum
Free Chlorine, ppm	2.0	3.0 – 5.0	10
Combined Chlorine	0	0	0.5
Total Bromine, ppm	2.0	4.0 – 6.0	10.0
PHMB	30	30 – 50	50
pH	7.2	7.4 – 7.6	7.8
Total Alkalinity	60	80 – 120	180
TDS	NA	NA	1,500
Calcium Hardness	100	150 – 250	800
Cyanuric Acid	0	30 – 50	***
Ozone			.01 over 8-hr time period

*** The proper level for cyanuric acid is in question because different states feel that this chemical can be dangerous; therefore, refer to state or local health departments for the proper guidelines. Testing on cyanuric acid does show certain health concerns, but these tests are limited to lab animals and cattle.

A level of cyanuric acid at 100 ppm and above will cause the sanitizers to lock up and slow down so much they become useless. Animals that drink water with that level of cyanuric acid develop diarrhea. In small children, there is an increase of ear infections. Older people tend to get weird rashes, especially in the genital area.

Problems with Spa Water

Certain things happen with water in a heated spa compared to the water in your pool. Your sanitizer depletes more rapidly due to the lack of reserves in a small quantity of water, especially when there are more people in the spa. The sanitizer itself has a shorter lifespan because of the temperature of the water. The reaction time of the chemical increases drastically as the temperature rises. Your pH has a tendency to rise due to temperature increases and the aeration from the circulation system and the blower. The pH will lower as more bathers are introduced because of their body oils and perspiration. This is a very good reason to keep your total alkalinity in check to prevent spiking.

Now that we have covered the appropriate levels of chemicals that will be present in your spa's water, this next chapter will cover the chemicals you will use to maintain proper water balance.

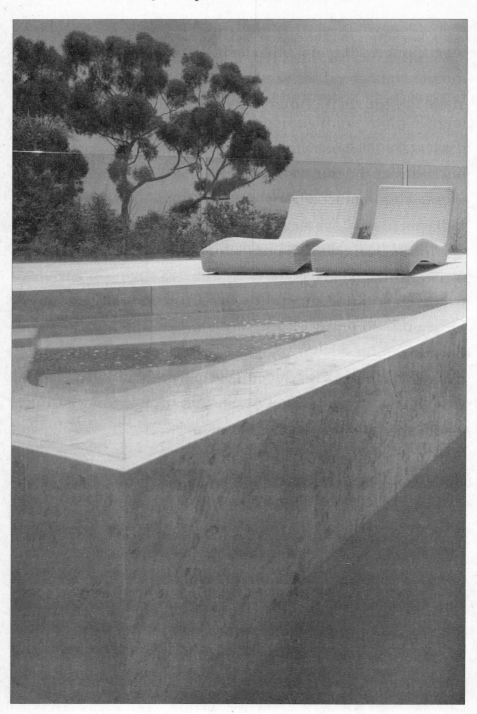

CHAPTER FIVE

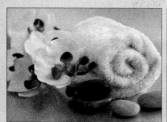 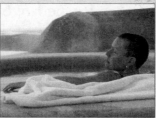 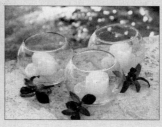

Chemicals and Cures

T his book will deal with the standard chemicals that are used on a daily basis by homeowners and professionals who take care of pools and spas. Many manufacturers make chemicals for spas that are diluted or buffered so you do not have to measure small measurements for dosages. This helps the homeowner, but when you purchase these chemicals, you will notice that they are still pretty pricey. You are paying top dollar for fillers and inert ingredients that are just adding more TDS to your spa. The charts that are included in this book are for regular industrial water maintenance chemicals and not special ones made strictly for spas. Buyer beware.

One of the purposes of this book is to make your experience enjoyable, safe, and inexpensive to operate without wasting money. This business of water maintenance cannot be learned totally from a book or even by taking a state test for operating a pool and spa maintenance business. This information is something that is learned over time. Experience is the real key for a person to become good at maintaining water on multiple pools.

For example, take the test for calcium hardness. The suggested levels for proper water balance are between 200 ppm and 400 ppm. If your water tests at 250 ppm, then there is no reason to adjust it because it is within a good range. But sometimes these franchise programs will tell a customer that they need to add calcium to get the level up closer to 400 ppm. Sometimes a spa owner is being sold a product that he or she really does not need, which happens all of the time. They way to avoid this is to test the water yourself. For comparison, it is okay to take a water sample in and see what they come up with. (Remember the difference the temperature of the water will make.) Knowing what is in this book and learning the way your pool or spa reacts to adjustments in chemistry will allow you to maintain your own water correctly.

Using pool chemicals requires you to read labels. Look for the amount of the chemical in the container versus inert material or fillers. Different manufacturers produce chemicals with different percentages of product. The best advice is to stay away from the large discount chain stores because sometimes these stores will agree with a manufacturer of some product to sell their product, which may have a different chemical compound than what you could buy from another store. Instead of a discount store, go to a pool store, and after reading the labels, make up your own mind on quality and value.

One great online source for spa products is Poolandspa.com (**www.poolandspa.com**). This company has been in business for 30 years, and not only sells supplies and equipment, but the management is also extremely knowledgeable. This Web site also offers a great array of additional information that will be useful to a spa owner, such as videos, articles, and a message board. Another great place to purchase spa products is from Hot Tub Works (**www.hottubworks.com**). In addition to a catalog full of various spa parts and products, this site also includes how-to videos, a blog, and an informational "toolkit." Spa Care Center (**www.spacare.com**) also offers a wide range of products. In addition, this Web site offers a live chat, an explanation of water chemistry, a troubleshooting guide, and an array of informational articles with helpful tips for the spa owner.

Sanitizers

Chlorine and bromine are the most popular choices for sanitizers. Other sanitizers include ozone, polyhexamethylene biguanide (PHMB), copper and/or silver ionization, and UV radiation.

Not only does chlorine act as a sanitizer, it also destroys microorganisms and acts as an oxidizer. Deodorant, suntan lotions, body oils, perspiration, pollen, dirt, and leaves are some of the things that a sanitizer has to deal with.

Microorganisms, such as algae, bacteria, fungi, protozoans, yeast, and viruses, consume chlorine because of **chlorine demand**, which refers to the amount of chlorine that will be needed to react with these contaminants before any chlorine is left un-reacted. Rain, wind, and humans introduce these microorganisms into the spa water. Most of these organisms found in pool water are harmless to pool users, but in a spa, they can make more of a difference because of the smaller water volume. Some are diseases and cause infection. These germs can be transmitted through water to other people who use the same water.

Harvard University concluded that one active adult swimmer loses two pints of perspiration per hour. Perspiration is loaded with compounds resembling the chemistry of urine. With the combination of these things as well as nasal discharge, fecal matter, and urine, you begin to realize why it is important to sanitize. These ammonia-producing items mixed with chlorine make **chloramines**, which are any combination of nitrogen or ammonia and chlorine. They control the release of chlorine and are slow to do so. Therefore, super chlorination — or what pool and spa technicians call **shocking** — is performed. This is simply the addition of an ample amount of chlorine, which breaks up the irritating chloramines and converts them back to chlorine. It also restores the water's clarity.

Quick safety note

All mentioned chemical elements are poisonous, depending on the dosage. Care must be taken when handling chemicals used to treat water. When dealing with water maintenance, a person who adds chemicals to a pool or spa is adding poisons to the water, just in a safe dosage. The proper dosage is very important.

Chlorine products and acid can kill. In April of 1915, the German army used chlorine gas against the French army at Ypres. The gas destroyed the respiratory organs of its victims, and this led to a slow death by asphyxiation. It was found that if the French army covered their mouths with a cloth soaked in urine — ammonia — it would have neutralized the chlorine gas. This tragic anecdote shows you how the effect of ammonia in the water can kill the chlorine and bromine in your spa. Chlorine and bromine do not mix with any acid or petroleum products. The results of mixing these items with anything can be very deadly. Pay extreme attention to these chemical warnings.

All manufacturers of chemicals are required to have Material Safety Data Sheets (MSDS) on all of their products. These sheets give information about the product, storage, fire danger, whether they are poisonous, and their chemical makeup. It would be a good idea to ask for a copy of the MSDS on the products you have at home for safety. In case of accidental poisoning, it would help the poison control center to know what the chemical compound is so they can correctly advise you on treatments.

Chlorine

There are many different types of chlorine for water maintenance, but for a spa there are only two types. Trichlor 1-inch tablets are perfect for a spa because of their size and because they can fit in the **feeder** — a tablet-dispensing sanitation device that is used for either chlorine or bromine — but they do have their limitations. Remember, chlorine starts to break down in temperatures above 85°F. Many manufacturers make tablets that contain 90 percent chlorine and the rest is stabilizer. (While spas normally do not need stabilizer if they are covered, this is how the tablets are made.)

The other type of chlorine is dichlor, which is in granular form, and works well for a chlorine shock. Those who are intent on having perfect control can use dichlor as a daily sanitizer.

Cyanurates: Trichlor and Dichlor

Cyanurates basically mean that cyanuric acid is part of the mixture and that the chlorine is stabilized. The two cyanurates are trichloro-trianzinetrione, called trichlor, and sodium dichloro-s-triazinetrione, called dichlor.

Cyanuric acid, which is commonly called conditioner or stabilizer, is a chemical used to minimize the decomposition of hypochlorous acid caused by sunlight in pools and spas. Cyanuric acid absorbs UV radiation. It can be a dangerous chemical if abused or mishandled and is considered a hazardous chemical. It can emit very toxic fumes of carbon monoxide, carbon dioxide, and nitrogen oxides. The dust from cyanuric acid can be explosive in certain quantities, and proper storage techniques need to be followed. However, cyanuric acid is not normally used in a spa, and adding any acid to this chemical can be very hazardous.

Trichlor

Trichlor comes in granular and tablet forms, which may also look like sticks. Trichlor is designed for the cooler water of swimming pools and contains a high percentage (90 percent) of available chlorine. Trichlor can be used in a spa but the high temperatures will cause it to dissolve very quickly. It comes in a 1-inch tablet, 3-inch tablet, a stick, cartridge, or granular form. It does have a long shelf life, and it is very slow to dissolve in cool water. This allows it to work extremely well in swimming pool floaters and erosion-type feeders.

Trichlor has a very low pH of 2.9 and requires frequent monitoring and pH adjustment to prevent damage to equipment and other metal parts. Trichlor is very slow to dissolve and is not recommended on the surface of a spa if it is in either the tablet for granular form.

Trichlor is manufactured by drying and cooling the sodium salt of cyanuric acid in the presence of chlorine gas. The resulting compound provides 90 percent available chlorine.

Dichlor

Sodium dichlor is the only granular type of chlorine that should be used in a spa. It is fast dissolving, will not cloud the water, is relatively pH neutral, and has a long shelf life. Because of its granular makeup, there is no way to automatically dispense it, and it must be added by hand. This is preferred to the small trichlor tabs because it can shock and sanitize the water. The drawback with dichlor is that you have to manually add the mixture if you are using it as the sanitizer. It is also more expensive than trichlor.

Sodium dichlor is chemically produced by adding soda ash and cyanuric acid to a solution of trichlor. When dried, the result is a granule that provides anywhere from 56 percent to 97 percent available chlorine, depending on the method of manufacture.

Bromine

The chemical name for the brominating tablets used in pools and spas is bromochloro-5, 5 dimethylhydantoin. You can see why they just call it bromine.

Bromine in true form is a reddish-brown liquid. If you look at the chemical name on the brominating tablets, you will notice "chloro" right behind the "bromo." That is because bromine needs chlorine or some other catalyst to activate it. By adding a little chlorine to the mix, you have a chemical that will activate when put in water. Normal bromine tablets are 61 percent bromine and 27 percent chlorine but this differs between different manufacturers.

Like chlorine, bromine produces amines called bromamines. Bromamines turn out to be far more carcinogenic than chloramines. Even trace amounts of bromine can trigger severe acne in sensitive individuals.

Although it is a good algaecide, there are some forms of organisms, most notably forms of either a black fungi or algae, that are resistant to bromine, and these bromine products will not kill them.

Although both chlorine and bromine are halogens, or salt-forming, bromine is more stable and less volatile in water than chlorine. Less of the bromine escapes the water as a gas because it has a very high evaporation point, which is what makes it so desirable in a heated spa.

Because bromine tablets already have their own oxidizer, which is chlorine, it is not necessary to use a separate catalyst. This combination makes hypobromous acid, and when joined with a contaminant, it becomes a bromine ion. The buildup of these ions in the water forms what is called a bromine bank. A **bromine bank** occurs when inactive bromine ions group together in a mass that can be reactivated when chlorine is added.

If a level of bromine ions of 15 ppm or more is present in the water, all the chlorine added is going toward converting bromide ions into hypobromous acid, and none of it will provide chlorine residual. That is why when you use sodium bromide as an algaecide, it eats up so much chlorine. Once the level of bromine drops below 15 ppm, chlorine can start to produce its own hypochlorous acid.

Most spas use bromine as the sanitizer. Some do not like the odor of bromine, but if used in combination with an ozonator, the levels of chlorine and bromine are reduced so you cannot tell if either is being used.

Bromine is more aggressive than chlorine, so managing your chemistry is essential to prevent equipment damage, not to mention unfavorable conditions that can occur for your body. If you have a low pH level in a bromine pool or spa, damage to metal is occurring. Bromine is not as forgiving as chlorine.

When talking with some pool and spa professionals, you probably would find that not many like using bromine. It is not that the product is inferior; some are simply afraid of it. When bromine is unstablized, it can react faster and more aggressively than chlorine. As a rule, the higher the level of bromine, the higher the pH is in the water. Because it is unstabilized, it dissipates when it is not being injected or eroded in the water. Therefore, pH fluctuates as the bromine dissipates.

To better illustrate this, here is an example: If you have a spa that uses a chlorine product that is stabilized and you test the water as the spa shuts off and remove the chlorine device, cover the spa for the night and retest in the morning. If you do this, chances are the level of chlorine will be the same as the night before because of the stabilizer. If you have a spa with bromine and test and remove the chemical device that feeds the bromine, cover and retest in the morning. You will discover that the level of bromine is lower than it was on the previous test. Even though bromine establishes its bank, it still will show a lower level, and it loses its ability to sanitize very quickly. You could add a catalyst and raise the level of bromine, but bromine levels do change fairly rapidly.

When it comes to the pH levels, they will vary depending on the manufacturer of the product and the amount of chlorine that is part of the chemical makeup of the bromine tablet.

When you decide what product you are going to use, try to use the same brand each time because different manufacturers' products can vary greatly. Another small piece of advice: Chemicals that are sold in discount stores usually have less of the active product in them, which is why they are cheaper. Always look at the labels. Spa chemicals are no place to cut corners to save a few cents on water management. When a product has less of the active ingredient, the manufacturers have to add fillers. These fillers can add to your TDS levels, and you may have to drain your spa more often. Pick a good product brand and stick with it.

When you first fill your spa, and every time you drain and refill it, it is a good idea to establish a bromine bank so the sanitizer will immediately start working in your spa. This is very easy to do. For a spa that has 250 gallons to 400 gallons of water, just add 1 ½ to 2 ounces of sodium bromide. This is called by many names — a popular brand is Yellow Treat®. Then you need a catalyst to activate it. Ozone can also activate the bromine, but the easy way to do it is to simply add 2 ounces of potassium monopersulfate to the water — the activation is immediate. Potassium monopersulfate is explained below.

Potassium Monopersulfate (PM)

Potassium monopersulftate (PM) is a free-flowing, white, granular solid that is soluble in water. It is present as a component of a triple salt including potassium monopersulfate, potassium sulfate, and potassium bisulfate.

The compound provides a powerful non-chlorine oxidation for many uses. Many pool and spa technicians use it for a shock in bromine pools and spas. They may occasionally use an algaecide for mustard and black algae that is called sodium bromide. It is a good algaecide for mustard and initial forms of black algae, but it needs a catalyst to activate it. Chlorine can be used, but for those people who do not like chlorine, then potassium monopersulfate is a good alternative.

For spas, PM should be added to spa water after every use at a dose of about 1 to 2 ounces per 250 gallons to immediately oxidize and eliminate organic contaminates that bathers introduce. PM eliminates many problems that can occur and keeps the water cleaner and safer. If the spa has an ozonator, then shocking is not needed after every use, provided that the system runs for a while afterward so that the ozone is circulated through the system.

Potassium monopersulfate is sometimes called shock and swim because it can be put into a spa and you can enter the spa 15 minutes later. However, it is better to wait an hour before entering a spa just to be safe.

PM does not break up combined chlorine. In a spa with bromine as a sanitizer, it activates the bromine ion, keeping it active long enough to oxidize the water. It oxidizes the waste products of the bathers and other organic contamination. Because bromine forms a bank, it can be activated over and over again by just adding PM.

Biguanicides

Polyhexamethaline biguanicide (PHMB) is its true name, but a common name for this substance is Baquacil. This chemical is expensive to use because it needs many supporting chemicals to do its job. It also reacts with different household cleaners, which can be dangerous when a spa owner cleans his or her spa and does not know what is reactive. If you choose to purchase this product to use in your spa, make sure you find an individual who has been trained and knows the product well. It will save you time, money, and plenty of frustration.

Additional Chemicals

When you purchase your spa or go to a pool and spa store to purchase chemicals, you will find a big assortment of items. A large amount of them are really not needed.

Spas are different than pools. In a pool, if you add a cup more of a chemical than what is required, it will usually recover. In a spa, if you add a teaspoon of something too much, it may ruin your whole water chemistry. When you deal with spas, you have to think in ounces, tablespoons, teaspoons, and sometimes grams. These measurements are very different than the measurements for a pool, where you think in pounds, quarts, and gallons.

Algaecides will not be discussed here because no spa should ever have algae. If your spa does get neglected and algae starts to form, simply shock the spa with chlorine, and when the algae is dead, drain your spa, flush the piping, clean the filters well after soaking them in a bucket of about 30 to 50 ppm of chlorine, and rinse the filters well. Proper filtration and sanitation will eliminate the need for algaecides and algaestats.

Soda ash

Also known as sodium carbonate, **soda ash** is a salt of carbonic acid. Most of the soda ash is made from table salt. It has many uses, but in pools and spas it is used to raise the pH of water. It neutralizes the acidic effects of chlorine and raises the pH of the water. The chemical formula of soda ash is Na_2CO_3. In a 1 percent solution, it has a pH of 11.3 but will not affect total alkalinity.

Sodium bicarbonate (bicarb)

Commonly called bicarb, **sodium bicarbonate's** chemical makeup is close to soda ash ($NaHCO_3$.) It is used to raise total alkalinity in water and has a limited affect on pH. The most common use of bicarb is baking, and it is also known as baking soda. The pH of sodium bicarbonate is between 7.9 and 8.2. If you use too much in a pool, the pH will not rise higher than 8.2. If you overdose a spa with bicarb, you can rapidly have scale form in pipes, on the surface, and on the equipment. When adding sodium bicarbonate in water, it is recommended that you mix it with water so that it is dissolved upon application.

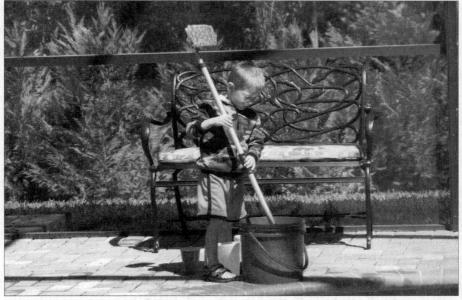

Figure 5-1 is Austin Shane mixing bicarb with water before adding it to a pool/spa combination. Courtesy of Dan "Grandpa" Hardy

Calcium chloride

Calcium chloride (CaCl2) is a combination of calcium and chlorine, and it is very soluble in water. It is used to raise the calcium hardness in water. It is an interesting chemical with many general uses, but what is important and should be remembered are the precautions that need to be used when dealing with calcium chloride. It reacts exothermically when exposed to water, which means it releases heat, and the chemical reaction that occurs can cause severe burns. When calcium chloride is mixed with water in a plastic bucket, the bottom of the bucket becomes very hot as well as the solution itself. Safety in storage must be taken because if a young child were to put some in his or her mouth, he or she would suffer burns. Facial protection and gloves should be worn when dealing with this chemical.

Chloramines

When chlorine is added to water, it generally forms hypochlorous acid, the powerful killing form of chlorine, and a hypochlorite ion, a relatively weak form of chlorine. The percentage of hypochlorous acid and hypochlorite ions will be determined by the pH of the water. As the pH goes up, more chlorine transfers from the lethal form to the weaker form. A general rule is that at a pH of around 7.2 the chlorine works at 80 percent, and a pH of 7.8 restricts the chlorine effectiveness to 20 percent.

Chlorine can combine with ammonia and nitrogen compounds in the water to form chloramines. By combining with ammonia and nitrogen, the free chlorine in the water is disabled. **Free chlorine** is the available chlorine residue that is not tied up with any other element that is available for sanitizing water. Chloramines are 60 to 80 times less effective than free chlorine and are formed any time ammonia and nitrogen are in the water. Bathers introduce some of the ammonia and nitrogen compounds into the water in the form of perspiration, urine, and saliva. Rain also introduces ammonia and nitrogen compounds into the water. Each drop

from hot tub to
SPA

photographs from the experts

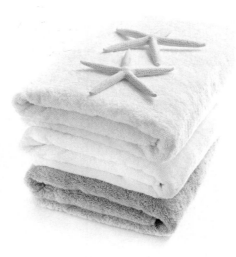

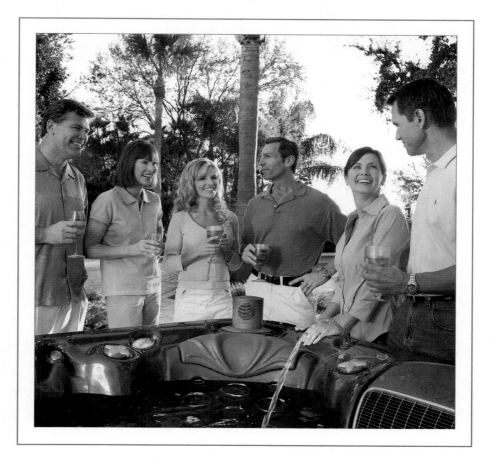

On the Assembly Line

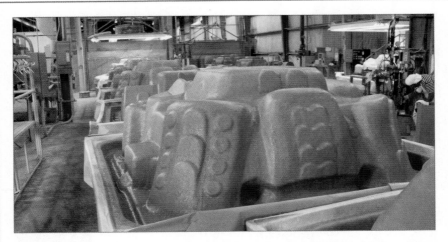

A view of spas at the Premium Leisure plant that have been molded and are ready for insulation jet installation.

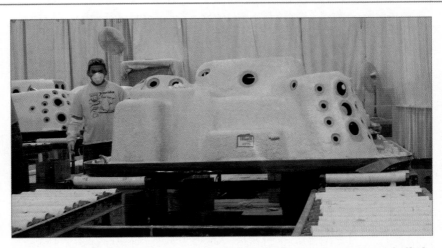

A spa with insulation on the bottom of the shell. The holes have been drilled into it so the jets can be installed.

Hot Tub and Spa Pieces & Parts

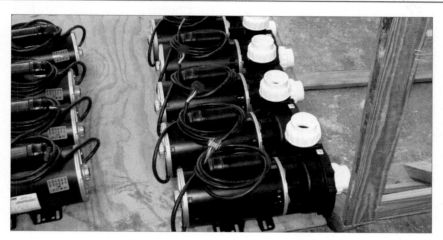

A group of circulation pumps, complete with PVC fittings and ready for installation.

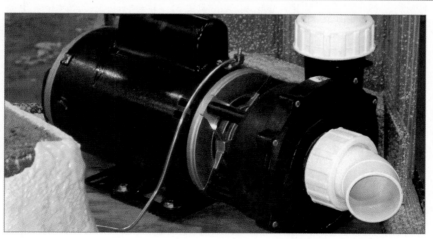

A close-up view of a pump installed inside the spa cabinet that is ready for hook-up. Notice the bonding copper wire attached to the motor. All equipment will be bonded to prevent electrolysis and heighten safety.

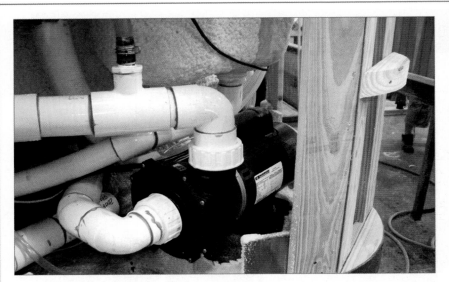

A pump installed in a spa cabinet and plumbed with rigid PVC.

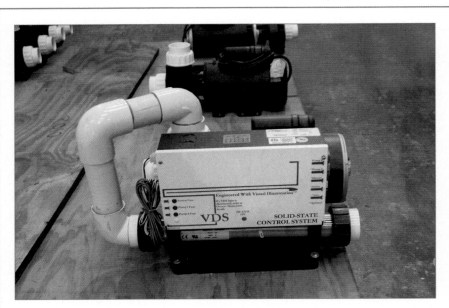

A pump attached yo a spa pack. The cylinder at the bottom of the spa pack is the heater.

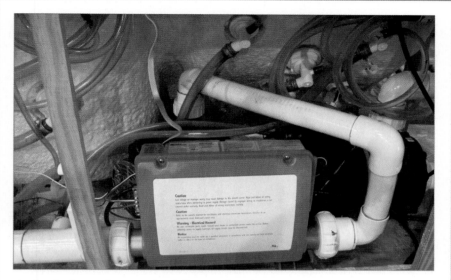

A plumbed spa showing the different clear lines that connect to the small jets.

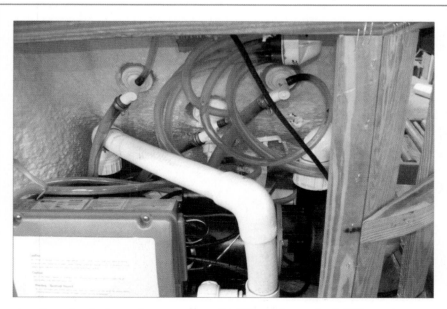

Another plumbed spa that uses clear, flexible tubing to feed different jets with water and air.

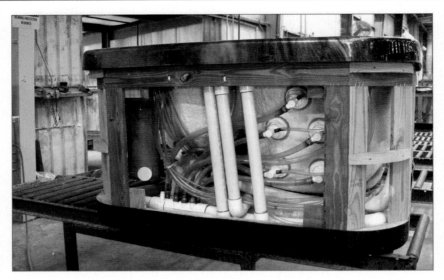

A spa that is plumbed and ready for cabinet installation.

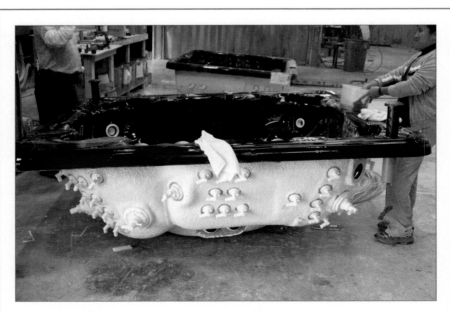

A large spa shell with jets installed that is ready to be placed inside the cabinet frame.

Interior

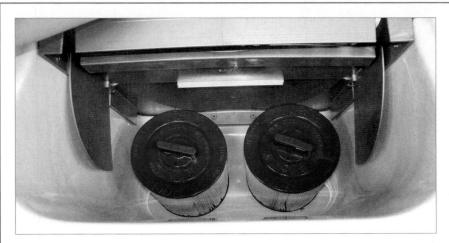

A dual-cartridge filtration system that has been installed in a spa.

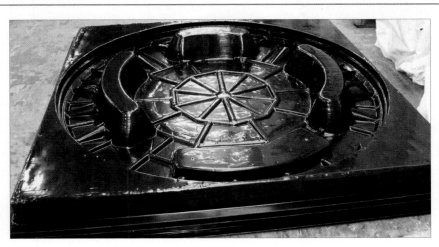

The molded bottom of a spa built by Premium Leisure. Using this molded base eliminates the lumber sitting on the ground and prevents wicking of the wood.

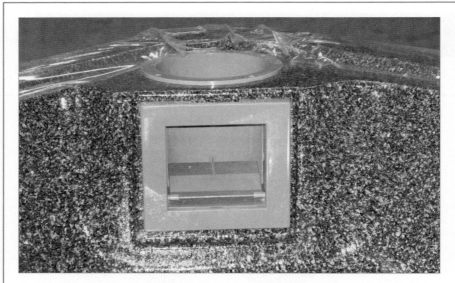

A skimmer installed on a spa with access for cleaning at the top.

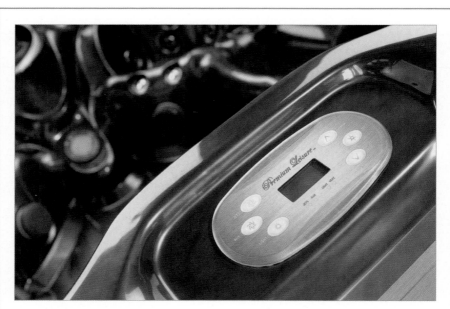

A digital control pad on a spa.

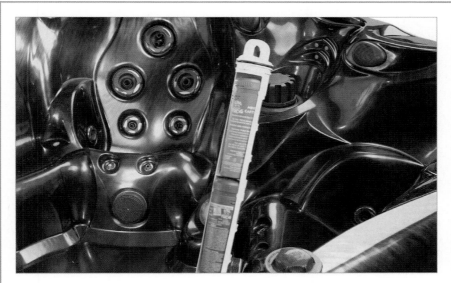

A set of jets used on a spa.

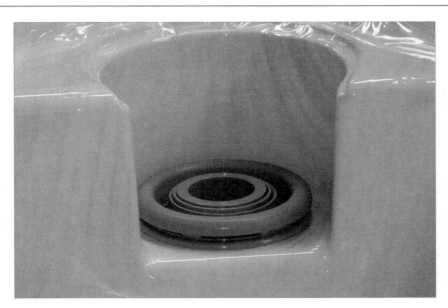

A floating weir skimmer installed in a spa.

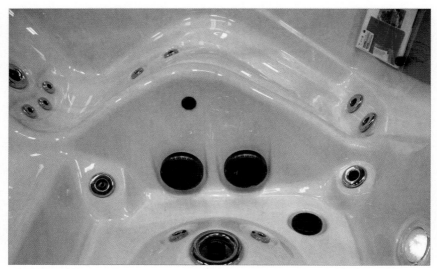

A lounge seat in a spa with the jets installed at key locations to massage different parts of the body. At the bottom is a jet pack that is used for foot massage or reflexology.

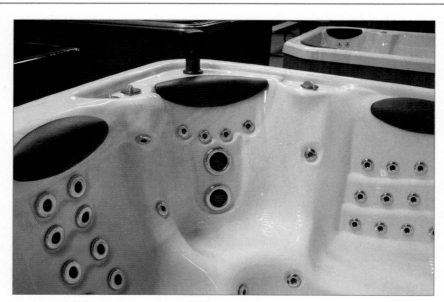

A view of different jet packs at different seating positions in a spa.

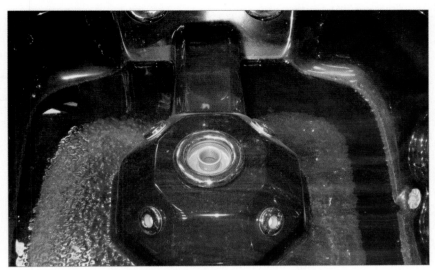

A jet pack that is used for massaging the feet. This can be used for reflexology therapy.

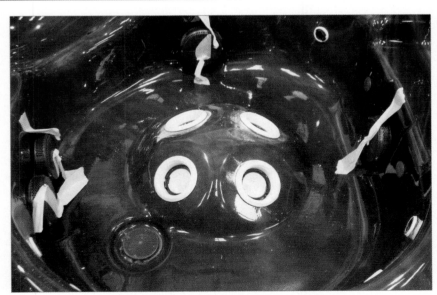

Another type of jet pack for massaging the lower legs and feet.

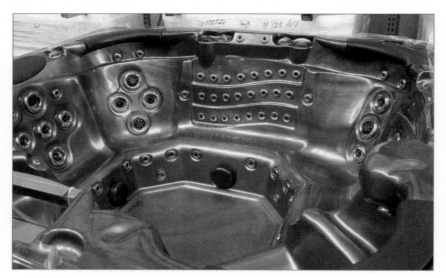

A large spa with different styles of jet packs installed at different seating positions.

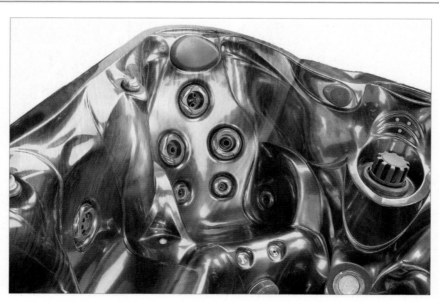

This seat position has jets to massage the back, the hip and kidney area, and behind the knees.

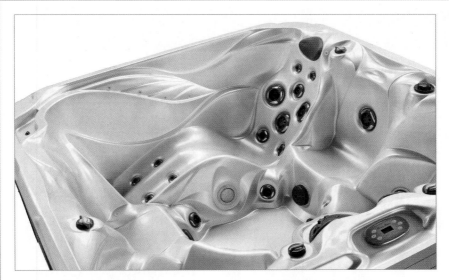

This spa includes different seating positions, jet packs, and a lounger.

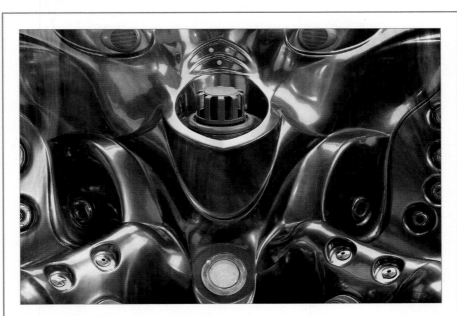

A spa with different jet packs and a center suction port.

Glamorous Hot Tubs & Spas

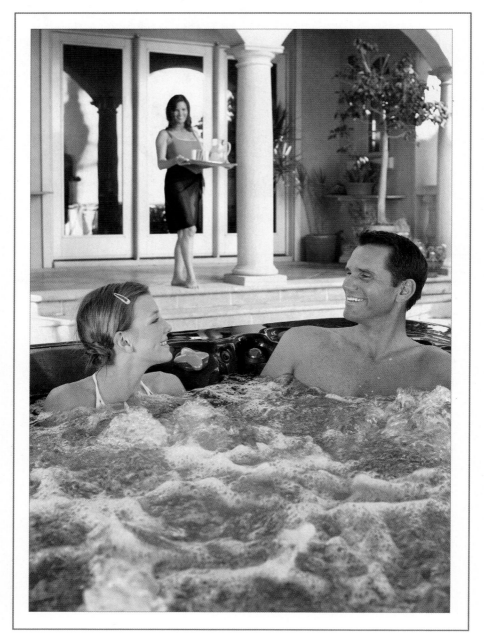

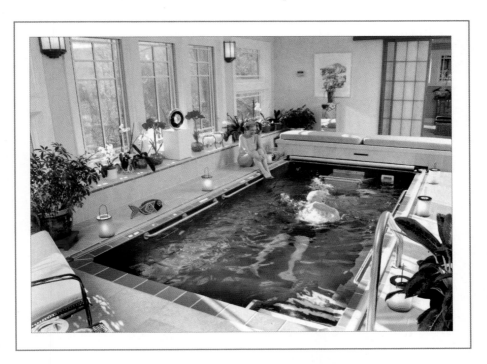

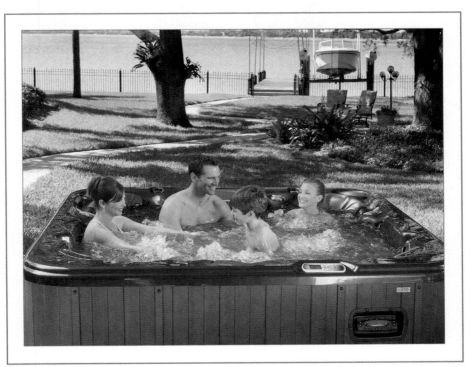

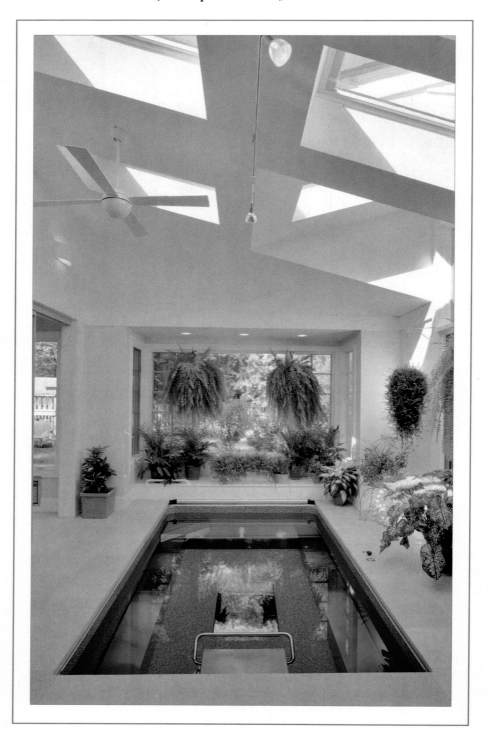

of rain has some dissolved nitrogen from the atmosphere, which is why your lawn looks so good after a rainfall.

Not only do chloramines smell bad, but they are also eye and skin irritants, and they can cloud the water. Another tip: If you smell chlorine in the pool, usually you do not have enough free chlorine and it is locked up, which makes chloramines. Shocking then needs to be performed.

If you take care of your spa by adding some PM to it after every use, you should not have chloramines or bromamines.

Alternative Treatments

Some spas have what some call a **metal ionization system,** which are commonly known as **ionizers**. They have an electrical charge that produces metal ions from copper, silver, or both that kills bacteria and algae when disbursed into the water. The problem associated with this is that while they may be successful disinfectants, they do not last or have any residual action. Also, they cannot reduce buildup from organic substances because they are not an oxidizer. When used in conjunction with a chlorine or bromine product, they are effective but not necessary. Whenever a metal is introduced in water, this metal will most likely cause surface staining. Ozone is preferred over these systems.

An important bit of information for you is that you will see chlorine-free products and systems that people will try to sell you. Beware of these products. Bacteria are monsters, and you must treat them accordingly. There is not a chlorine-free product that takes care of water's needs. Some products may work on a short-term basis, but eventually you will need a better sanitizer than what they present as the ultimate cure. In heated water, bacteria are going to grow without the best sanitation available, so why risk it to save a few dollars? Usually, these "miracle cures" for water wind up costing you more money than if you were using the traditional methods of either chlorine or bromine.

Defoamers

A defoamer is a product that reduces the bubbles that look like — and sometimes are — soap. Mostly, the soapsuds come from makeup, body oils, detergents that were not rinsed out of your clothing, and other contaminants. It is important to remember that a defoamer is not a product that keeps working over and over again. After two to three applications, it is time to change the water.

Enzymes

An **enzyme** basically eats up lotions, oils, and other organisms that normally clog the filter. The water line that usually has deposits of these unwanted items attached to the spa does stay cleaner when using an enzyme. This is one of the chemicals that you do not search for by price; purchase it by brand name.

Clarifiers

A **clarifier** is simply a product that attracts small particles in your water and makes them larger so that the filtration system can remove them. When purchasing a clarifier, it is important to make sure it is not also a flocculate. A **flocculate** is something you add to a pool that combines particles in the water, causing them to sink to the bottom of your pool or spa where they can easily be vacuumed. Some clarifiers turn into flocculates, depending on the dosage. Too much of the product and the particles attract each other, and because of their weight, they drop on the floor of the spa. Pick a clarifier that is not a flocculate, such as SeaKlear®. It is an all-natural product, and if you overdose, it does not flocculate.

Scale and metal remover

Treated water in a spa really should not need this unless you have metals in the source water. Whenever you are aware that you have rust, iron, or any other metal present in your water, when you fill your spa, you can use a **Bobbie**. This is a sock that attaches to your water hose and acts as a filtration for metals and other contaminates. This will remove metal from the initial fill. If needed, you can use a metal out or scale remover to aid in the removal of these particles if you have bad water. Scale should never occur in a spa with properly treated water, and when you cannot control it easily, then drain the spa.

Saltwater Spas

A saltwater spa is simply a spa that has a chlorine generator installed on it. It is not seen on many portable spas, but many pool and spa combinations are salt-generated systems.

The system is a very simple but somewhat expensive piece of equipment. Water that has been treated with salt to a specific level flows through a container, or cell, and with an electrical current that produces chlorine. It can be regulated by how long the cell is active during the time in which the pool or spa runs.

When a person gets out of the salt water, they will notice how good their skin feels. It is like being in a bath with Epsom salt. Your skin feels soft, and because you are actually in a mild saline solution, it is less irritating to your skin and eyes than the traditional chlorine that you are used to. Manufacturers of these pieces of equipment claim that it is healthier than traditional methods of sanitation. Usually, a person that is considering converting his or her pool or spa to salt is easily persuaded when they actually swim in water that is treated in this way.

Now that you know the chemicals you will need to maintain the proper water balance in your spa, it is time to get in and start enjoying your spa. This next chapter will show you the different forms of therapy you can use in your spa.

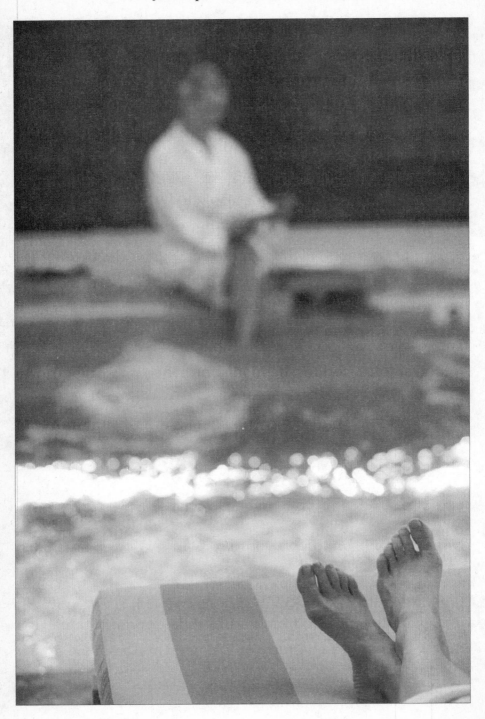

CHAPTER SIX

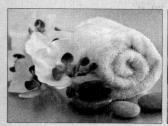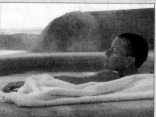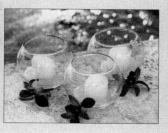

Therapy from Your Spa

There are many different types of therapies that you can use in your spa or hot tub. The list can be quite long, but this chapter will deal with some of the more common types of therapy. If you are interested in one of these therapies, you should research it well to see if that is what you are after.

There have been an increasing number of studies concerning the health benefits of hot water healing. Although there are many things that affect your body in hot water, the two that are most discussed and researched are heat and buoyancy. They are what create the healing and relaxation of hot water.

Hot water raises your body temperature. The blood vessels that are closest to the skin dilate, improving the blood circulation by cutting the resistance of smaller vessels.

During this increased temperature, your body releases endogenous opioid peptides, which are primarily endorphins (the natural chemical in the body that makes you feel good). When endorphins increase in the body, they help strengthen the immune system. It is also reported that they improve sleep, help prevent headaches, and give you more energy.

When your body is first introduced to hot water, it reacts by increasing your heart rate, which brings additional blood to the surface to help cool the body. When your heart rate increases and the blood flow increases, it brings an increase of oxygen, white blood cells, and different antibodies, which in turn revitalizes the blood cells. Initially, your blood pressure increases, but once the blood vessels dilate or expand, the resistance is reduced on the heart and your blood pressure will lower.

Sebastian Kneipp, who some consider the father of hydrotherapy, performed many studies involving hot water therapy as treatments on different diseases. He found that water has the power to dissolve diseased matter, and it removes the diseased matter from the body. As the body cleans itself, it actually strengthens because of the cleansed blood, which delivers clean oxygenated blood to the body, aiding the tissues and maximizing circulation.

In addition to the affect on diseases in the body, Kneipp found that extended immersion in hot water actually encouraged a natural process of the body to detoxify through increased sweating. Toxins will actually be eliminated through perspiration and lymphatic drainage.

The following is a case study from a spa owner who has been using her spa for therapeutic purposes. Aside from the increase in endorphins and the dilation of blood vessels, this spa owner discovered her spa helped her with another physical condition.

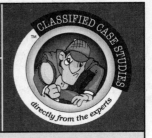

CASE STUDY: SPA OWNER
KATHY MCEVOY

During the last 15 years, I have owned two spas, both of which were purchased at a large-scale retail store. I was very pleased with the first spa I purchased, and when it had to be replaced, I purchased a second spa at the same retailer for about $3,500.

I have scoliosis and use the spa for therapeutic reasons about four nights a week. I enjoy having a spa with targeted jets and different seats that target different areas of the body. If a spa is being purchased for therapeutic reasons, this is important. The spa also should be easy to get into and out of. It is also important to consider where the spa will be located in your home, thus ensuring it is easy to access — especially in the winter months, which is personally my favorite time to use the spa.

My spa gets cleaned once every six months, and sometimes the water is changed out in between cleanings. The spa also has an ozonator, and there have never been any problems with the water.

How Water Aids in Repairing Your Body

Many people exercise on a regular basis, and when you work out, your muscles develop microscopic tears. When a muscle tears, it allows waste such as lactic acid to build up in the affected muscle. This is what causes muscle fatigue and soreness. As these tears repair themselves, the muscle actually becomes stronger. When people overwork themselves, these small tears become larger, allowing more lactic acid to build in the muscle. This causes more discomfort and pain. Hot water can actually help heal these muscles by increasing the blood flow to the damaged areas and help carry the lactic acid and other metabolic waste away from the muscles, which eases fatigue and makes the muscles relax.

When the muscles relax, the pressure is lowered to the surrounding nerves and vessels, which brings natural pain relief. In the case of joint pain, the relaxation of the muscles causes them to become more limber by providing a level of resistance that assists in rebuilding muscle strength and supports the damaged joint or muscles surrounding the sore joint.

The *Journal of Rheumatology* did a study on the effectiveness of hot water therapy on treating back pain. The study was devoted to lower back pain. The group that was used to study lower back pain was broken into two groups. One group only took medication for relief, while the second combined medication along with hot water treatments. After a period of three weeks of hydrotherapy sessions, the group involved in the water treatments noticed a measurable difference in pain intensity and duration and had more flexibility. After six months, the hydrotherapy group showed a significant improvement, which led to the decrease of the use of medication.

The Mayo Clinic has recently conducted studies and found that patients soaking in hot water that had suffered strokes, traumas, and other injuries actually benefited from warm water therapy because it reduced blood pressure. This treatment was found to help rehabilitate the participants from these illnesses and let the patients exercise in the water when they may not have been able to do so normally.

A study by the *New England Journal of Medicine* has proven that the regular use of a hot tub or spa will simulate exercise by increasing the heart rate because hot water mimics the same physiological effects of exercise. Unlike regular exercise, the use of water decreases blood pressure instead of making it rise and stay there for a time. By doing this, the added circulation means better digestion.

This study was conducted for three weeks, and scientists noticed that those who stayed in a hot tub for 30 minutes a day for six days a week lost about a pound per week. The average weight loss was just less than 4 pounds for the three-week period. Regular use of hot water also reduces the appearance of cellulite. The increased circulation reduces fluid retention and relieves swelling, which decreases the appearance of cellulite.

The National Swimming Pool Foundation (NSPF) funds many studies about hot water immersion. In December 2007, a report conducted by Dr. Bruce Becker in Colorado Springs, Colorado, was released. Co-funded by the NSPF and Washington State University, the study presented its findings first at the 2007 World Aquatic Health Conference in Cincinnati, Ohio.

This report claimed that warm-water immersion had a significant effect on the autonomic nervous system. It showed enhanced balance between parasympathetic (relaxation) and sympathetic (stress) components of the nervous system. The studies tend to show positive health-related implications. Details of further research have not been released at the date of this printing.

Individuals who suffer from post-traumatic gonarthrosis (a disorder of the knee joints) have showed significant results from hydrotherapy. Aquatic exercises for women suffering from the symptoms of menopause can help if they have bone density issues. There is evidence that people suffering from chronic obstructive pulmonary disease (COPD) find benefit while doing deep breathing exercises in a spa. The steam opens the airways, and exercising promotes overall physical fitness.

It has been said that athletes that use hydrotherapy actually increase their endurance and running performance. The Department of Physical Medicine and Rehabilitation at the University of Vienna has also found that hydrotherapy can play an important role in the treatment of primary varicose veins. With patients that have undergone major abdominal surgery, the Southeastern Louisiana University School of Nursing found that hydrotherapy could help alleviate pain and assist in wound healing.

Helping You Sleep

The National Sleep Foundation (NSF) encourages people to establish a regular routine of relaxing by soaking in a hot bath or hot tub while reading a book or listening to soothing music, as this promotes sound and deep sleep. Over 70 million Americans suffer from sleep disorders, according to the National Institute of Health (NIH). As you get less sleep, you develop more stress.

Sleep deprivation is believed to have many adverse effects, including nervousness, grogginess, memory lapses, depression, and erratic mood swings. The dangerous part of the lack of sleep is that many of us revert to other means to get to sleep. The number of sleeping aids is increasing, whether over the counter or prescription drugs. This does not cure the problem, but instead makes you depend on something else that is not good for your body.

After a good 15-minute soak in hot water, your core temperature rises slightly. When you get out of the hot water and you continue to relax, within 90 minutes, your core temperature will start to drop and it tells the body it is time to go to sleep. When this happens, you will fall deeper into a restful, revitalizing sleep.

Safety and Health Issues

This cannot be stressed enough: It is highly recommended that you check with your doctor before using hot water, steam, or any other heat-related therapy. Here are some of major health and safety issues to be aware of in relation to spas:

- It is highly advisable to limit or restrict alcohol consumption as well as drug use while using a spa.

- Drugs that relax muscles or make you relaxed or dizzy may not react well with hot water, and the chances of falling asleep are greater when using prescription or recreational drugs. These drugs, along with alcohol consumption, will increase your chances of passing out in the spa and drowning.

- Pregnant women should absolutely not get into a hot water spa without first consulting with a doctor. A person that normally has low or high blood pressure, heart disease, diabetes, blood disorders, or lung problems must seek the approval of a doctor and must start with lower temperatures and work his or her way up slowly.

- For those hot tubs that are heated by firewood or other uncontrolled sources, the temperature must be monitored, and it is recommended that you do not go over 104°F. Drowning is the primary cause of injury concerning a hot tub. Going over this recommended temperature, as well as extended stays in hot water, can lead to heat stroke, heart attack, skin burns, and even brain damage.

- A child should never be left alone and unsupervised in a hot tub, not even for a minute. An adult may choose to gamble with his or her life by enjoying the hot water while drunk or on some drug, and that is his or her business. But an unattended child left in a hot tub is inexcusable.

Above all, use common sense when using your spa.

The Dangers of Hot Water Treatments

As with all good things, there is a bad side to hot water therapy. This section shows you what can happen when your water is not properly treated and sanitized. Maintaining your water is important and never should be taken too lightly. Before entering and after exiting a hot tub or spa, taking a shower is very important.

People who are suffering from a bacterial infection, a viral infection, fungi, or parasites should not use a spa that other people are using. This is the problem with public spas. Using a spa that a sick person has just used can transmit some communicable diseases because bacteria thrive in heat and water. Maintain your spa regularly, and when in doubt, drain out the old water, sanitize, and refill.

There have been studies that show that the fertility of males may be decreased with regular use of hot water therapy. In 2007, a study headed by Dr. Paul J. Turek of the University of California–San Francisco revealed that exposing men to hot baths or hot tubs could lead to male infertility. The effects can sometimes be reversible.

In a study of hot water immersion, it was found that hot water can impair both sperm production and mobility. The small test consisted of 11 patients who were exposed to repeated hot water soaking and were asked to cease this activity for a minimum of three months. After that time, 45 percent, or five patients, responded favorably to the cessation of heat exposure and experienced a mean increase in total motile sperm counts of 491 percent after three to six months.

This is not unusual. In Japan, there is a century-old practice that barred childless men from conducting business deals in hot tubs due to its believed effect on fertility.

An important point when talking about treating injuries and certain problems is that heat sometimes makes injuries worse and ice should have been used instead of heat. Always seek medical advice if you have an injury that is more than just the normal muscle soreness that occurs after a workout. With some injuries, heat actually promotes swelling.

For those who are interested, the NSPF has opened up a blog called the Aquatic Therapy Blog, found at **www.aquatictherapist.com**. It deals with many issues that may be important to a spa owner.

The following case study details a woman who uses her spa regularly to soothe aching muscles after athletic activity. Her experiences are similar to many other spa owners who purchased their spa to use for rehabilitation purposes.

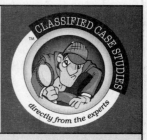

CASE STUDY: SPA OWNER CLAUDIA

Beverly Hills, California

I have always loved spas. I bought my spa new for about $2,500 and use it almost every night, sometimes during the day as well. I use my spa for recreational and therapeutic reasons. The spa comes in handy after I play volleyball, and I even use it before playing to stretch my muscles. Sometimes it is great to use for relaxing after a game or just having friends over to enjoy the soothing water.

To keep my spa clean and running efficiently, I clean the filter every month and change the filter every few years. I clean the water periodically with a skimmer to remove dirt, leaves, and pine needles. My spa has a cover because I think it helps keep the water hot and clean. I also add regular chlorine tabs once a week to keep the water balanced.

I think spending time in my spa is the greatest. I think there is nothing like being outside in nature — whether it is hot or cold — with the trees, stars, and critters.

Hydrotherapy

Hydrotherapy is one of the oldest forms of treatment known to man. It involves using water to soothe pain and disease treatment as well as using water for healing purposes. The warmth of the water, the buoyancy the water provides, and the turbulence of the water aids in reducing pain, faster recoveries after some surgeries, stress relief, and the reduction of some spasms and discomfort. This treatment is best known for sports injuries, neck and back pain, arthritis, and knee injuries.

In the early 1700s, written works were published on the subject of hydrotherapy, formally called hydropathy. From there, testing and using warm water continues to this day. There is also a therapy association for dogs for ortho-related injuries and surgeries.

Hydrotherapy has many different forms. There are the regular baths, packings, hot air baths, compresses, and many more. Some of the first explanations of hydrotherapy have been traced back to around 1,500 B.C. Hippocrates used hydrotherapy a great deal to treat many illnesses and injuries around 400 B.C.

One of the advantages of water is that it absorbs more heat for a given weight than any other substance and is an excellent conductor of heat. Water has the ability to change states from boiling hot water to ice, making it a perfect therapeutic agent. In the vapor state, it is perfect for aromatherapy.

Different water temperatures can produce different therapeutic effects. A temperature variation of only 2°F can totally change the therapeutic effect. Because this book deals with spas and hot tubs, this section will concentrate on the full or partial immersion bath type of therapy. Normally, these will be within a temperature range of 100°F to 104°F for up to 20 minutes. Longer periods are not recommended for the elderly, young, anemic, or anyone who may have a tendency to hemorrhage. Before doing hydrotherapy, please consult your doctor.

Heat can transfer from one object to another through conduction, convection, or conversion. **Conduction** is when energy flows from an area of higher temperatures to an area of lower temperatures; **convection** occurs when energy is transferred into or out of an object by the movement of a surrounding liquid; and **conversion** happens when one form of energy transforms into another. The heating and cooling effects of hydrotherapy produce the conduction of heat from the water to the body.

Hydrotherapy stimulates the endorphins, which helps control pain and relieves tension. Pain relief comes from the bubbles the jets and blower produce. They relax the muscular tension and reduce swollen joints, which in turn reduces pain. Hydrotherapy helps improve circulation and helps remove toxins from the body. Regular use of hydrotherapy helps your immune system control viruses, bacteria, and infections. It is also believed you can improve your complexion by removing toxins through your sweat glands.

To achieve healing in the body, good blood flow is essential. Blood needs to be well oxygenated, rich in nutrients, and low in toxins. The effects of hydrotherapy are perfect to achieve this effectively.

The most important way you can use your hot tub for therapeutic reasons is by using it to break up the stress cycle of everyday life. Stress is related to many health issues and some severe physical and psychological problems. Some conditions that stress is associated with include high blood pressure, digestive problems, insomnia, depression, and anxiety attacks. Stress also hurts the immune system.

When you are under stress or in pain, your body goes through some chemical changes. During these changes, your blood pressure and pulse rate increase, which in turn can lead to other health problems. Regular use of your spa can slow down the stress reaction and helps you relax and unwind, which helps a person deal with the pain that they have.

As a general rule of thumb, after the first five minutes of bathing, your blood pressure and pulse rate decrease. After ten minutes, the circulation in your hands and feet improve. After 15 minutes, your muscles start to relax, making the muscles more pliable. When muscles are relaxed and you stretch, lactic acid and others toxins are more easily released from your body.

Moores Cancer Center at the University of California–San Diego has done research on cancer patients and concluded that hydrotherapy is thought to promote wellness and optimize overall health. In their research, they use a combination of warm and cold water, ice packs, humidifiers, and liquids to combat dryness and dehydration, steam, and colonic irrigation.

The American Cancer Society reported, "Hydrotherapy is an accepted, useful form of symptom treatment for many ailments. The ability to promote relaxation in its many forms is well established." They are talking about external forms of hydrotherapy. The internal types of irrigation will be left to physicians.

The fear or danger of hydrotherapy is not from the treatment itself, but can come in the form of bacterial diseases from contaminated and unsanitized water, especially water that is found in public bathing facilities. This is another reason to learn proper water maintenance.

The more you use your spa, the more improvements will be seen. It should also be said that the type of spa you own matters a great deal on the effect of the treatment. Optimal water movement, circulation, and jets that concentrate on different areas will greatly affect the results that one is after.

Reflexology

Reflexology is simply applying deep massage to the feet or hands, which in turn affects corresponding parts of the body. The major benefit of using reflexology is the reduction of stress in different parts of the body. In other words, by massaging a certain part of the hands and feet, it can stimulate corresponding parts of the body using the nerves of the body. It is believed that the feet and hands are broken up into zones that correspond with other parts of the body through the nerves.

Think of the nerves in your hands and your feet like the wires that run through your car. They go from one control or area to another control or area. There are maps of the nerve areas, just like a wiring schematic, to know where to massage to affect a certain area of the body.

Reflexology, like some of the other therapies, has been practiced for thousands of years throughout Asia. In 1913, Dr. William H. Fitzgerald showed that if you apply pressure to a certain area, it could have an anesthetic effect on another area. That was the first known introduction to reflexology into the United States. Eunice Ingham mapped the entire human body into reflexes on the bottom of the feet in the

1930s; she found that certain pressure points corresponded with each organ in the body.

During treatment, the bather feels relaxed, so relaxed he or she may even fall asleep. You may develop a tired feeling with some tingling sensations. Your body temperature may slightly reduce itself, being in such a state of relaxation.

After using reflexology, great stress relief and deep relaxation have been reported. You develop improved circulation, and you have more energy in a relaxed state. As with the reduction of stress, your immune system will also become stronger.

A great deal of emphasis is being placed on not substituting medical treatment for reflexology. As with many types of therapies, some people can become too dependent on a particular therapy. Reflexology is not a cure for a problem but an aid in helping manage certain age- and injury-related problems.

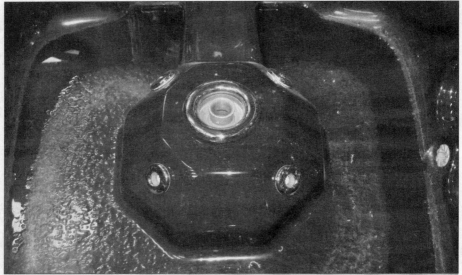

Figure 6-1 is a foot jet system in a spa used for massaging the feet. Courtesy of Premium Leisure

Aromatherapy

Aromatherapy has been around since the early days of man. Smell affects the body in that if it is a pleasant smell, it tends to relax you. If a skunk sprays you with his scent, however, that definitely will raise your blood pressure. The sellers of the body oils used in aromatherapy tend to over exaggerate some of the effects to sell their product. Aromatherapy usually will not cure problems but will instead manage or alleviate the symptoms these problems may cause. If it does nothing other than relieve a little stress, it is a good therapy and does have health benefits.

Aromatherapy is inhaled from the mist coming off the spa. The best time to use aromatherapy is when the water is hotter than 100°F and the outside temperature is cold. The colder the outside temperature, the more evaporation, which means more vapors are available for you to inhale.

When a particular oil or fragrance is added to hot water, it is enhanced by the temperature of the medium that it is being put into. Hot water tends to make the smell stronger and opens up your sinuses more, allowing you to breathe in more. Many spa owners enjoy the therapy, and if it is pleasant, then it relieves stress. As stress is relieved, then other health ailments may disappear. When this occurs, then the therapy has worked.

The following is a list of oils used for aromatherapy. This is not a complete list of oils used, but it shows the essential oils and what they can be used for. Please note that the author and publisher are not responsible for the misuse of any of the following oils. Only a practicing aromatherapist can advise you of the safety of the oils. Each oil needs to be investigated depending on the manufacturer for its strength, dosage, and proper use. As with chemicals used to treat the water in your hot tub or spa, more does not mean better and can be dangerous. Always follow the directions supplied with the oils you purchase. Information supplied on the Internet is not always accurate, so always consult the manufacturer's specification sheet for the product.

Below is a list of the more common essential oils and the ailments they can be used to treat.

- **Angelica** can be used for coughs, colds, fevers, and to help with indigestion.

- **Aniseed** can help with indigestion, bronchitis, and coughs.

- **Balsam of Peru** is used for colds, bronchitis, hemorrhoids, bedsores, rashes, eczema, stress, and asthma.

- **Basil** is used for colds, fatigue, migraines, depression, and nausea. It can also help with concentration.

- **Bay** helps with colds, insomnia, and rheumatism and can be used as a decongestant.

- **Benzoin** is used for coughs, arthritis, and itching and can be used as a mild sedative.

- **Bergamot** helps with acne and stress, relieves tension, and functions as an antidepressant.

- **Birch** can be used for rheumatism, ulcers, and eczema.

- **Black pepper** is helpful for treating acne, pains, rheumatism, and can offer cold relief.

- **Cardamom** can be used for colic, coughs, halitosis, headaches, heartburn, indigestion, fatigue, stress, vomiting, constipation, gas, and nausea.

- **Carrot seed** can help treat eczema, psoriasis, ulcers, and some gout.

- **Cedarwood** helps treat acne, bronchitis, and lung congestion.

- **Chamomile** calms nerves and helps with insomnia, asthma, hay fever, nausea, diarrhea, and fever. It also has anti-inflammatory effects and can serve as a disinfectant.

- **Cinnamon** aids circulation, improves heart and digestive tract functions, helps spasms, and can be used as an antiseptic.

- **Citronella** acts as a deodorant, stimulant, and insecticide.

- **Clove** is used to remedy toothaches, digestion problems, asthma, nausea, and tension. It can also be used as a sedative or an antiseptic.

- **Coriander** can fight against the flu, indigestion, rheumatism, and nervousness.

- **Corn oil** can be used to soothe your skin.

- **Cypress** can remedy menopausal problems, circulation, colds, nerves, hemorrhoids, and whooping cough.

- **Eucalyptus** can be used as an antiseptic, diuretic, analgesic, and can also treat ulcers, skin infections, and rheumatic aches and pains.

- **Fennel** helps the digestive tract, menopausal problems, obesity, constipation, and nausea.

- **Fir** is used to help with asthma, arthritis, bronchitis, colds, coughs, flu, muscle aches, and rheumatism.

- **Frankincense** relieves nerves, tension, bronchitis, stress, colds, and respiratory problems.

- **Geranium** can help with menopause, diabetes, throat infections, and uterine and breast cancers. It can also act as a sedative.

- **Ginger** relieves muscle aches and pains and can help with colds and nausea.

- **Grapefruit** can assist with liver problems, migraines, and has been known to help in drug withdrawal treatment.

- **Jasmine** can help depression, menstrual problems, anxiety, and enhances relaxation.

- **Jojoba oil** is used for psoriases, eczema, acne, and even hair care.

- **Juniper** can help the nervous system, digestive problems, acne, and fatigue.

- **Lavender** can be used as an antibiotic, antidepressant, sedative, and antiseptic; can help relaxation; and can relieve tension, insomnia, asthma, arthritis, and headaches.

- **Lemon oil** can be used for insect bites, tension headaches, digestive stimulation, and wrinkles.

- **Mandarin** helps with nervousness, liver problems, and anxiety.

- **Neroli** can be used as an antidepressant, aphrodisiac, antiseptic, digestive aid, sedative, and can help with bacterial infections.

- **Nutmeg** can relieve vomiting, muscle aches, arthritis, nervousness, and insomnia.

- **Orange** can be used for depression, anxiety, constipation, nervous conditions, and muscular spasms. It can also be used as a sedative.

- **Parsley** can help with nervous conditions, kidney problems, and menstrual and menopausal problems.

- **Patchouli** can be used to help treat stress, wrinkles, dandruff, hives, fatigue, and acne.

- **Peppermint** helps in digestion, respiration, and circulation. It also helps remedy fatigue, gas, the flu, migraines, and liver problems.

- **Pine** helps the bladder, kidney, chest infections, fatigue, the flu, muscle pain, sore throats, and colds.

- **Rose** can help with menopause, dry skin, gingivitis, stress, insomnia, inflammation, hay fever, asthma, eczema, and nausea.

- **Rosemary** assists muscular conditions, sprains, depression, fatigue, memory loss, and migraines.

- **Sandalwood** can treat scars, bronchitis, acne, diarrhea, insomnia, stretch marks, and sore throats.

- **Spearmint** helps indigestion, intestinal cramps, fevers, and colic.

- **Tea tree** can be used to help with insect bites, acne, asthma, colds, flu, dandruff, warts, diaper rash, and coughs.

- **Red thyme** eliminates whooping cough, warts, and fatigue.

- **Valerian** can treat insomnia, rheumatism, backaches, bruises, menstrual issues, colic, stress, and migraines.

- **Lemon verbena** can treat indigestion, heart palpitations, bronchitis, stress, and insomnia.

- **Vetiver** helps anxiety, nervous tension, and insomnia, can relax muscles and acts as an antiseptic.

- **Ylang-ylang** can be used as a sedative, antiseptic, aphrodisiac, and can help high blood pressure, intestinal infections, impotence, and depression.

This seems like a long list, but in reality it is a shortened version. The main thing to remember is that each essential oil may have different effects, depending on what part of the plant it comes from and how you personally will react to it. Knowledge of the product that you purchase is important.

When you research oils, you will find essential oils and base oils. The essential oils are the fragrance oils and the base oils are the carrier oils that some essential oils need to work properly.

Some of the therapies are like a good recipe, and one needs to pay attention to the mixture because some are relaxants and sedatives. Too much in hot water may cause you to fall asleep or pass out, which could be deadly.

Watsu

Watsu is a body massage while in warm water. This allows for the body to be stretched and manipulated in more ways than if a person were lying in a bed or on a massage table. This therapy may not be possible in some of the smaller personal spas due to the lack of space.

Watsu is fairly new to the therapy community. It was created in the early 1980s by therapist Harold Dull, who, at the time was the director of the Harbin School of Shiatsu and Massage in Northern California. In larger pools, they sometimes incorporate three other techniques: waterdance, healing dance, and the Jahara technique.

More information on Watsu and these other techniques can be found on the Worldwide Aquatic Bodywork Association Web site (**www.waba.edu**) and the Aquatic Bodywork in Australia Web site (**www.aquatic-bodywork.com.au**).

Therapy Options Overview

Today, the Internet is a good way to research these therapies, and you will find that the information on these four therapies is very extensive. Hydrotherapy is the most widely recognized and openly used therapy out of the ones covered in this chapter. Along with these four therapies, there are many others that you may want to investigate. Trying an alternative therapy is a personal decision. Keep in mind that as with all treatments and therapies, they are not quick and take time. Just like taking some medication, therapies have to be used for a while to take effect.

Different forms of water therapy are options you should consider when selecting a spa. Different spas have packages for some of these therapies, and if you are interested in one or more of these therapies, then it is beneficial for you to know about them before you purchase a spa. Other than learning how to maintain your spa properly so that you enjoy it to the fullest in a safe and healthy manner, learning about therapy options is equally as important. If you choose not to use any of these therapies other than the hydrotherapy and if you purchase a spa with different therapy options, you have wasted your money. Put your money in the options that you wish you use.

This next chapter will cover all the equipment and switches you will need to be familiar with should you want to use your spa for therapeutic uses or for recreational uses. It is important to know how to use the features properly so you know how to maintain them and what functions they serve.

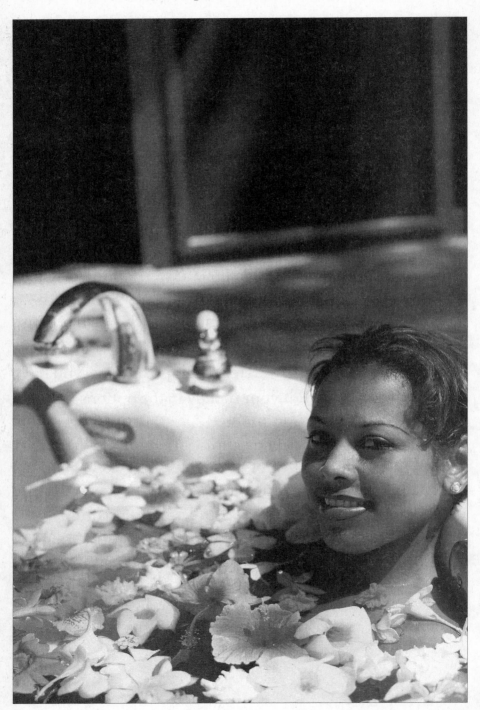

CHAPTER SEVEN

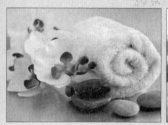 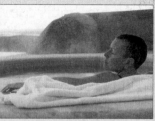 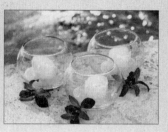

Other Equipment and Controls

While you have already been introduced to the main components of the spa, there are other pieces of equipment you should be familiar with. Some are self-explanatory, but others require a bit more explanation. This chapter will describe the various controls and accessories your spa may include.

Air Buttons and Switches

An **air button** is a simple device that was designed for safety and is relatively inexpensive but works well. An air button is used to control blowers, lights, and jet pumps. It is a simple button mounted in a housing that is either mounted into the surface of the spa or located close to the spa if it is not a portable version.

The air button activates an air switch mounted on the motor of a pump, blower, or light. When you push the button, it forces air through a small hose that is connected to the switch on the intended device. This switch can have only one function or multiple functions, eliminating the need for the spa user to come in contact with electrical switches. They come in many different shapes and sizes.

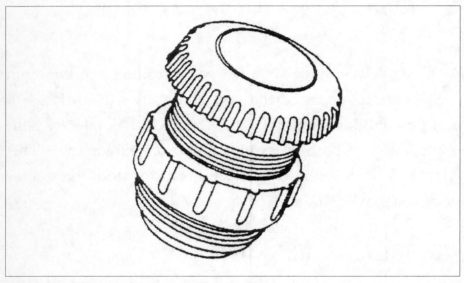

Figure 7-1 is a simple air button. Courtesy of Premium Leisure

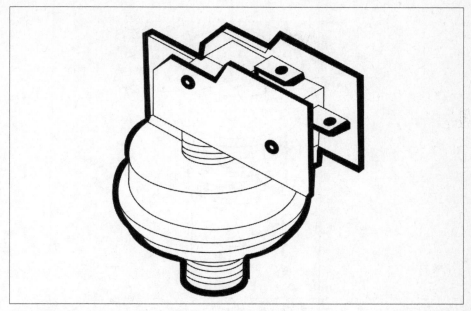

Figure 7-2 is a typical pressure switch. Courtesy of Premium Leisure

Air Controls

An **air control** is also a very simple device that allows you to regulate the size of an opening. It controls the amount of air that can go to certain types of jets or functions to make them more or less aggressive. They vary in size, depending on their function, and are also mounted on the spa surface top.

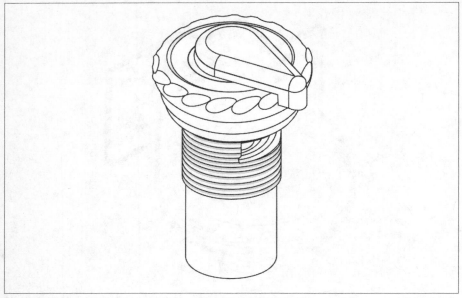

Figure 7-3 is a typical air control valve. Courtesy of Premium Leisure

Control Panels

A **control panel** is the pad mounted on the spa that lets you turn on your different devices, usually by pushing a button or a touch screen. The different styles and types of control panels are endless and can perform a couple of simple functions to multiple complicated features. They are matched with the spa packs to allow them to activate the right equipment.

The older units had a dial that functioned as the thermostat for the heater. The newer ones are digitally controlled, and the thermostats are located in the spa pack or other locations under the spa.

There are spa-side security panels that have codes that need to be used to activate the spa, and some can be located away from the spa in restricted locations. These were all designed with safety in mind.

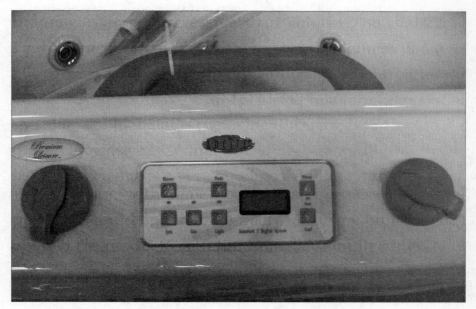

Figure 7-4 is an electronic control installed in a new spa. Courtesy of Premium Leisure

Lights

Lights for a spa come in many shapes, sizes, and colors. On permanent spas, fiber optic lighting can be used to make the experience quite enjoyable.

You can purchase lenses that can snap onto your light to change color and set the mood. The right light can make the experience very relaxing and pleasurable. After all, it is the relaxation and therapy that you are after.

Stereos and Televisions

CD/MP3 players and flat screen televisions have been added as extra features for some spas. There is no problem with relaxing in a nice massaging body of water while listening to some music that helps relax and relieve stress. After all, whatever it takes to get rid of the daily stress is beneficial. However, there is a problem with the televisions in the spas.

With music, one can sit and relax in the spa and, when finished, get up and leave the spa after the session. When a television is part of a spa or even in the same room as the spa, the spa user has the tendency to stay for a long time watching a show or movie. Extended periods in hot water is not a good idea because it can be unhealthy.

Short intervals in hot water are beneficial, but when one stays in for an extended period of time, it can cause a stroke, heart attack, and even brain damage. The point to hot water therapy is not to raise the core temperature of your body to dangerous levels; while it can vary depending on the person and his or her health, the general rule of thumb is not to spend more than half an hour in temperatures higher than that of the human body. The other danger that applies to people with heart problems or high blood pressure is that once they leave the hot water after a very long time, their blood vessels may not constrict fast enough and could cause their blood pressure to drop, which can make them pass out.

The other reason not to stay in the spa for long periods of time is because while you are in there, you are breathing the mist or steam coming off of the water. The more of this you breathe, the higher the chance of getting hot tub lung from the bacteria that may be in the steam if your spa's water is not cleaned properly. Some symptoms of hot tub lung include coughing, shortness of breath, weight loss, and fever. People suffering from the disease can also experience fatigue, and the oxygen levels in the body can fall so low they may need to be put on oxygen. The disease is often misdiagnosed as asthma or bronchitis. You can prevent this disease by ensuring that you keep your spa water clean and sanitary, preventing the growth of the bacteria that cause hot tub lung.

After reading this chapter and the previous chapters about the different elements of your spa and what features they offer you, you will need to know how to properly maintain your spa. The next chapter will cover all the maintenance you will need to perform to keep your spa running at its best.

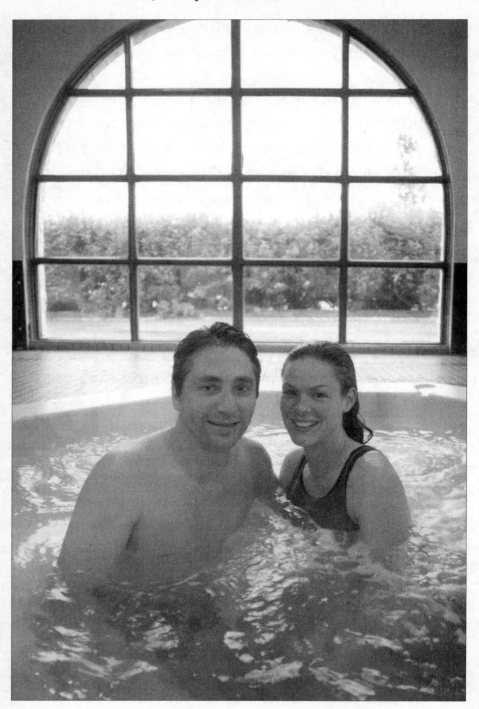

CHAPTER EIGHT

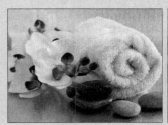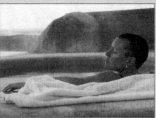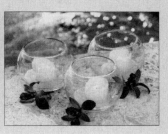

Cleaning and Maintenance

One may think that because a spa is smaller than a pool, it would be easier to clean and maintain. Depending on the circumstances of the bather load and how the bathers address the issue of using a spa, it can be more work than a pool. This part of the ownership of a spa, as well as the chemistry, requires commitment and consistency. The risk factors involved in a spa that is not taken care of can be dangerous in several ways.

Before examining the actual act of cleaning and maintaining your spa, you should have a general idea of the equipment needed to do the job properly. This next case study provides a little more insight to what one spa owner does to keep her spa running effectively.

CASE STUDY: SPA OWNER DEB BAILEY

Arkansas

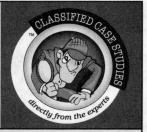

I purchased my spa online from a major television shopping network for about $700. I have a bad back and my husband works construction, so we use it for therapeutic and recreational reasons. We use the spa more in the spring and summer months and do not use it during the winter months.

My husband is the one who primarily performs maintenance on our spa. He changes the filter once a month, and we add chemicals almost daily. We also use a spa cover to keep our water clean because we live near the woods and frogs will lay eggs in our spa if we do not use the cover. We do a pH balance test and algae tests daily and use chemicals like chlorine from a large-scale retail chain. One difficulty we have encountered with buying our chemicals from a large-scale retailer is they do not carry the chemicals during the winter months here, so we have to purchase a larger supply before winter begins.

We recommend purchasing a portable spa like we did because you can purchase them at a cheaper price and get accustomed to owning a spa. These kinds of spas take more work sometimes, but they are also plenty of fun for the whole family

Test Kit

The test kit is one item that you should not be cheap on. Generally, you can expect to pay around $20 for a good test kit. There are many kinds of test kits, including DPD test kits, kits that have tablets, powders, OTO kits, and also test strips. Once you get used to a certain item and it works, stick with it. The specific brand of testing kit you choose is not important; the important part is that you choose one that tests for your sanitizer, the pH, and alkalinity. Calcium and stabilizer are optional on a spa unless you are using water from a water softener or using a stabilized chlorine product for sanitation.

Telescoping Pole

The telescoping pole is what your tools attach to — the brush, the vacuum, the net, or the leaf rake. This pole can be made of metal like aluminum or fiberglass. For a spa, this pole does not have to be very long; it just needs to be long enough to easily reach all areas of the spa. Poles come in many lengths and usually are two pieces that are adjustable. Some utilize an internal cam to tighten and lock the pole in place, and others have an outside cam that tightens a big nut to secure the pole.

Leaf Rake

A leaf rake that is used on a portable spa is a little different than the ones you use in a pool. The spa leaf rake, which resembles a net, is smaller and is made of a smaller micron mesh that removes the smallest particles floating in a spa.

If used correctly, it can remove some oils and lotions. It can become saturated just like a cartridge filter and needs periodic soaking in a cleaning solution of dishwater soap with enzymes.

Corner Brush

A corner brush is a small, round brush that fits on your pool pole and is about 4 inches in diameter. It is perfect for those tight corners and hard-to-reach dead spots in a spa. It is made of mostly nylon bristles. Do not use a metal bristle brush in a spa except for the concrete models. It also is good for cleaning around the different jets and water features of a spa.

Spa Brush

A spa brush is smaller than a standard 18-inch pool brush and varies in size, depending on the area of the spa the brush is for which it is to be used. These brushes are also made of nylon bristles. They, too, are used to clean the floor and walls of a spa and are also good to take the scum off the water line of the spa.

Sponge

A sponge is another tool you will want to use for your spa. You may want one with a fine scrubbing pad attached to the other side. Sponges are useful tools for cleaning the scum that deposits on the spa at water level. They are also perfect for cleaning oil off the spa with the soap that the manufacturer recommends for the spa. Care must be taken not to damage the surface of a portable spa, and no abrasive cleaner should be used on a fiberglass or acrylic spa.

Spa Vacuum

A spa vacuum suctions small debris from the water. There are numerous spa vacuum manufacturers. One popular vacuum is the Spa Wand, manufactured by Polaris®. It has a hand-pulled shaft that creates suction and picks up almost everything off the seats and floors of a spa. It also has a removable screen to catch debris that needs to be taken out of the water. These items may be a little pricey, but they are well worth the money. If you cover the screen with a piece of panty hose, it will filter out some of the smallest pieces.

Spa Leaf Vacuum

A spa leaf vacuum is like its larger brother you use on a pool; it suctions larger debris from the water. This vacuum is powered by water and has a water hose that is attached to the vacuum that forces water through small holes in the center, pointing upward and creating a vacuum. The debris is forced through the opening in the cleaner and deposits the debris into a removable bag. You may want to put a piece of nylon hose over the outside of the bag to allow the bag to hold debris smaller than the normal micron rating of the bag. The micron rating refers to the particle size a filter can remove; the smaller, the better.

Cleaning Products

This is an area that gets some people into trouble. First of all, if soap has been introduced into the spa and water is flowing rapidly, the suds that it would produce would surely make any clothes washer jealous. The soap gets into the plumbing and is very difficult to get out. Do not use the wrong cleaning compound for a portable spa. Make sure you use a product approved by the spa manufacturer to clean the surface of any spa, including an old wooden tub. Never use an abrasive cleaner in a spa unless it is a pumice stone in a concrete spa. Using an abrasive cleaner can damage the spa's surface, and once the surface is damaged, it is difficult and costly to repair.

Concrete model spas can be cleaned just like a pool, and some are plumbed with a cleaning port to vacuum the spa using the filtration system to catch the debris. If it is a self-contained unit that never flows into the pool, make sure you choose your cleaning product wisely. The nice thing about a concrete spa with an exposed aggregate finish is that a quick wash with trisodium phosphate (TSP) takes care of the soap and oil problem; follow that by flushing the surface and plumbing very well. Then once you have it drained, you can do a quick acid wash on it to remove any minerals that have deposited on the surface.

To acid wash your spa, you will need to use muriatic acid. This chemical is a skin, eye, and respiratory irritant, so it is important that you follow all safety precautions when using the acid — be sure to use rubber gloves, protective eye goggles, and a chemical dust mask or a respirator. Also follow any precautions on the product label. Mix a solution of ½-quart of muriatic acid and 1 gallon of water in a bucket. Using a scrub brush, start on the inside floor of the spa and work your way out of the spa while washing. Be careful not to splash the solution on your face or clothes. Rinse the spa thoroughly and allow it to dry completely before refilling the spa.

A spa with a cover needs to have the cover cleaned and protected using whatever product the manufacturer recommends. The area between the cover and top of the spa also needs to be cleaned and free of any obstructions that may prevent a good seal.

A good deal of evaporation occurs with a spa. The water level in the spa is critical for the proper performance and water filtration. The spa's bather load will affect the water because more bodies in the water displaces the water, and the water loss will be greater with many people in a spa than if there were just one or two. Remember, it is important that you maintain the proper level of water at all times. You will find out that if the proper level is not maintained and you turn on the spa jets or blower, standing beside the spa may make you a very wet camper. If a jet has a non-restricted area to flow water, it will be forceful and shoot a long way. A good way to judge the correct level of a spa is to turn it on. If the water shoots out of the spa, chances are the water level is too low. Also, if the level is low and you have a floating weir skimmer, that could suck in air and cause the pump to lose prime and possibly damage the pump and plumbing.

Periodically remove the access panel and inspect to see if there are any leaks — this is usually found on the front under the control pad where the equipment is located. Usu-ally, algae growth is a good sign that something is leaking. If you notice a seal leaking in a pump, have it repaired. If there are any other leaks, make sure they are repaired also. A small amount of moisture underneath the cabinet can cause damage and result in unhealthy mold and mildew.

When you drain your spa, it is a good idea to take the hose and force water through all of the jets to help remove debris and water that could not normally flow out. This is extremely important if you have had your spa sitting without water in it for a while because as water sits, bacteria and algae will grow. You may want to take a spray bottle with a mild chlorine mixture and spray it in each nozzle to let some sanitizer help keep these problems from growing. It may seem time-consuming, but it will be worth it when the time comes to refill your spa.

Once you fill your spa, it is important to shock the water before using your spa to kill the bacteria. This procedure needs to be done with chlorine or bromine. A non-chlorine shock will not kill the bacteria and other little items that have grown while the spa was sitting empty. During this procedure, it is a good idea to leave the cover off your spa so the air will be able to carry away the bacteria that is in the mist coming off the spa. When you shock your spa, you must remember that when high levels of chlorine or bromine are used and the pH is low, the water becomes very aggressive and can damage surfaces and your equipment. This is where some thought has to be given to prevent damage.

The best advice for refilling a spa that has sat empty for a while is to refill with clean water and shock it. Before you shock it, make sure your pH level is in the range of 7.4 to 7.8. Remember that whatever product you choose to use for a shock will affect the pH. The sanitizer needs to stay active for at least four hours to be able to do the job. At the end of the four hours, drain the spa, flush it, and then refill it.

Upon refilling your spa, make sure that your filters are clean and free of all the junk that hopefully was trapped during the shocking period. If you are going to use bromine, establish a bromine bank.

Before doing this, make sure that your water balance is within the proper parameters, and then establish the bromine bank by adding 2 ounces of sodium bromide and 2 ounces of chlorine for spas under 400 gallons (or 1,512 liters). If you are using chlorine, raise the chlorine level to 5 to 8 ppm. Turn the spa on and let it run for a few hours. Once you have done this, you can retest the water and make adjustments to your balance. Let it run normally for a day and retest. Once the parameters are in line with proper balance and sanitation, it is safe to use. Always check for leaks after running a spa that has sat empty for a period of time.

Even when you are careful, you may end up making a big mess by spilling water while cleaning your spa. This is something to keep in mind when you are deciding on where your spa will be located. In the middle of your carpeted living room would not be the best choice, for instance.

Air locks are common in spas and are caused when air is trapped in the lines and equipment. Some spas have bleeder valves to help eliminate this problem, but sometimes they do not work properly or completely. Your manufacturer should have a section in the operator's manual that covers their type of spa. If you have an air lock where the pump runs but you have no circulation, there is something that you can do.

First, make sure that your heater is not on until you are sure the spa is running properly. Many spas do not have flow or pressure switches that keep the heater from operating in case of limited water flow. This means that the heater can burn up pretty quickly because of overheating.

If you have a spa with only one circulation pump, it is easier than if you have multiple pumps. On the top of the pump or pumps, there is a union fitting. These fittings are designed to be tightened by hand because using a tool can break the plastic fittings. They have an O-ring that is between the two parts of the union that seal. Make sure to loosen it just a little so that the O-ring does not come out of the groove that it sits in. With water in the spa, make sure the power is turned off to the spa and loosen the union nut. Air and water should come out, and you may see air bubbles coming out of some of the jets. This is what you want to see so that the air is purged from the system.

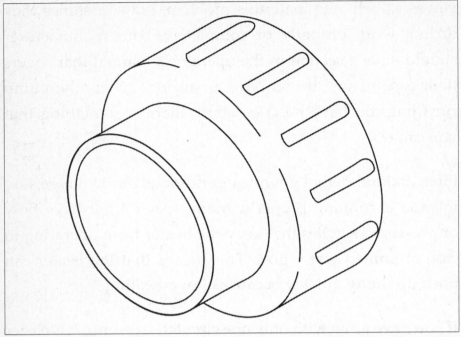

Figure 8-1 is a standard union nut found connected to a circulation pump. Courtesy of Premium Leisure

Your spa should have a slide shut-off valve on both sides of the pump. You can close them, loosen the union nut, and open the slide valve so that the water loss is minimal but adequate. Once this is done, it is recommended that you let the spa sit for a while and allow most of the water to drain off the components. When satisfied, you can turn the power back on and turn on the spa. If you still have a flow problem, you are going to have to bleed some more. If it runs properly, turn on all pumps to make sure all the air is gone from the system.

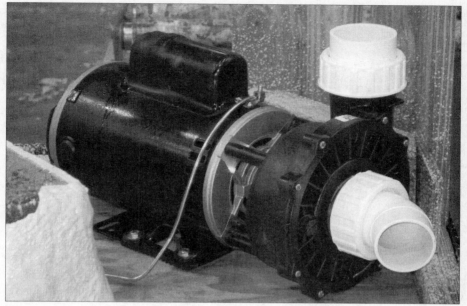

Figure 8-2 is a mounted pump with union nuts installed. Courtesy of Premium Leisure

Your spa needs to be properly protected with a GFI switch. Standing in water around your spa and having electricity turned on to your spa can be dangerous if it is not installed properly. If your GFI has a trip button, trip the breaker to make sure that it works properly. If it does not trip, call an electrician before you proceed further with using the spa. This should be done from time to time to make sure it is working properly. If you live in some areas such as Florida, ants will move to a piece of equipment that has electricity flowing through it, and these pests can mess up many things such as switches, pumps, and motors.

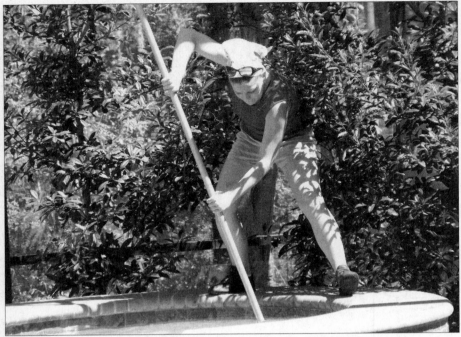

Figure 8-3 is Marcie cleaning the walls of a permanent spa. Courtesy of Premium Leisure

After reading about the maintenance of a spa and what you will need to keep your purchase running like new, this next chapter will assist you when you decide you want to purchase a used spa.

CHAPTER NINE

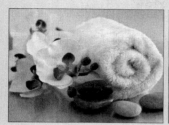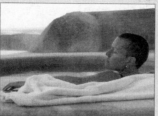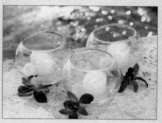

Purchasing a Used Spa

You may decide that you would like to own a spa but really would not like to fork out all the money it costs to buy a new spa. Buying a used spa can save money, but you have to know what you are doing and the possible dangers that are involved with this.

Before You Buy a Used Spa

Buying a used spa is no different than buying a used car. Insist that you see it run before you buy it. A person who is moving is usually the best choice to buy a spa from. These families usually are forced to sell their spa because it is too difficult to move it long distances. It is also a good idea to hire a spa technician to take a look at the spa before you purchase it. The Internet is not a good place to find a spa because a spa or hot tub should not be purchased without seeing it in person first.

If you talk with the spa owner and he or she says the spa has not been run in a long time, there is a chance that equipment has deteriorated. Normal weather effects can corrode electrical components that have just been sitting idle. Seals and O-rings will be dried out and damaged. The other thing to think of with a spa that has been sitting and not used for a period of time is the water that was left in the lines is full of bacteria and other dangerous things. Algae that has formed in the lines of a spa may be difficult to get rid of.

A spa that has been sitting in freezing temperatures can have damaged plumbing and equipment from the water that is trapped in a spa and is not drained properly. When the water freezes, it expands with force and will crack lines and pump housings.

If the shell of the spa has been exposed to sunlight for a period of time, the surface may have blisters on the acrylic layer and even unseen damage that may remove the lamination from the fiberglass underside and the reinforcing product.

A spa that is set up and running is the only spa to consider when you are looking for a used unit. Here are some things to inspect when looking at a used spa or hot tub:

- Naturally, the shell is important to examine to see if there are any problems that are noticeable. Be careful to look for small cracks or fractures in the surface. Even though some of these cracks and fractures may be fixed easily, some may not be easy to repair and may require a shell replacement to cure the problem.

- With the spa running, remove the inspection cover and look inside using a flashlight. Look to see if the shell is separating or if there are any noticeable leaks. Physically feel the lines to see if they are hard and brittle. Look carefully at the frame and the cabinet to see if there is mold or evidence of wicking and rotting of the wood.

- If you are not going to hire a professional to inspect the spa, turn off the power and remove the cover from the spa pack. You are looking for corroded connections. Look for wires that have evidence of overheating and are discolored.

- Sometimes a leak will seal itself temporarily, so look for any evidence of a previous leak, such as stains on the wood or calcium and sanitizer deposits at the site of the leak. Also check for the insulation that is under the spa.

- During operation, make sure the spa-side controls cover all functions and do what they are suppose to do. Ensure that the speed controls work as well as the heater, thermostat, and lights. Check all the air valves to see if they change the flow of water when opened and closed.

- Ask for the original spa manual that came with the spa. Not only will it help you check the operation of the spa, but it will also give you information on service centers and warranty. Some warranties are transferable.

- Listen to the pumps. There should be no whining or grinding during operation, and you can put your hand on the motor of the pump and feel if there is a vibration.

- Remove and inspect the filter(s) to see if maintenance has been done regularly on the spa. A totally plugged filter may indicate that the owner was not too concerned with maintenance. The filtration system is the heart of the spa as far as maintaining water.

Once you have picked out the spa that you want to purchase and have had it delivered, the next thing you should consider is your spa's location. Where you place your spa should be a key component to the type and size of the spa you would like to own. Several factors come into play in this decision.

Location: Indoors or Outdoors

When considering installing your spa inside the home or inside an enclosed area, some things need to be addressed that are very important. When installing a spa inside a home, the first thing you need to consider is whether the spa will be able to fit through the door or opening it needs to get through to be placed indoors or in the enclosed area. Most spas will not fit through a doorway, either because they are too tall or wide, or the height of the spa may be too wide to fit through the door.

The importance of ventilation

Another factor to keep in mind for an indoor spa is ventilation. A spa's location must provide good ventilation for several reasons. First, the bacteria that can form in the lines and surface of a covered spa are waiting to come out and greet you. When you open the cover for your spa, you should let it sit open for a while so that spores and debris can be blown away from the tub. Before entering the spa, you should turn on the jets and let them circulate for a few minutes to help sanitize the bacteria that have been dormant in the lines and equipment. Breathing the mist or vapor from initially opening your spa, especially if it has not been used for a while, can be very bad for your health. If not properly ventilated, the emission of the chemicals used is in the air, and the bathers are breathing them in as well.

The other good reason for good ventilation is that if it is located in a room that is made of wood or sheetrock, mold and mildew will build up, and this can be a very costly thing to get rid of — not to mention the health effects on the people in the home.

Providing sufficient drainage

The next point to consider is if the area has drainage. From time to time, you will have to drain your spa, and the water has to go somewhere or have access for a water hose to direct the water to where you want it to go. Also, standing water that results from using your spa — whether it is spilled, overfilled, or from the evaporation during use — will form algae and bacteria and has to be dealt with. This is another good reason for good ventilation. The location needs to be one where you can clean the area and may pressure wash it to remove buildup. The spa water does not need to be contaminated by things on your feet when you walk to the spa.

Reasons for not choosing an enclosed location

Enclosed areas for spas are not preferred for several reasons. The main reason is the health danger that can be associated with the enclosed places. Recently people have become seriously ill, and some have died from being exposed to bacteria and some viruses associated with hot tubs.

Another important factor to consider is what your spa going to sit on. Think about this for a minute. Water weighs 8.33 pounds per gallon (ppg). A basic portable spa can weigh up to 600 pounds, and then you have the weight of the bathers in the spa. The danger of putting a spa on a wood deck is an issue. It must be built to withstand the weight, the abuse of being wet, and the chemicals that can be absorbed by the wood. Cedar is a good wood for this purpose, but it is best if you have a deck built with treated lumber developed specifically for decks.

The location of a spa must be strong, level, and capable of supporting the weight. It needs access to electricity to make the spa run properly and must be provided with all the safety features installed. A certified electrician familiar with installing spas needs to do that job.

The spa must be located in a place where the homeowner or service person has full access to service and is able to maintain the spa. Even if your spa has an access panel, it is usually only for certain access to the spa pack and the drain and valves. Plumbing extends all around the spa, and space needs to be left to remove panels and provide full access to the entire spa. If your spa has a wood cabinet as previously described, you have to be able to access your spa to maintain and clean it. These decisions will make life much more pleasant for you in the long run.

If your spa has to be hardwired by an electrician, it would be advisable not to fill the spa until it has power to it. There is no need to start bacteria growing in a new spa without being able to circulate and sanitize the water.

It is strongly advisable that before you fill your spa you designate one person to adjust the water chemicals in the spa because having two people playing with chemicals is an accident waiting to happen. The next thing is to sit down and read the manufacturer's instructions on the spa before doing anything. Do not always trust what the salespeople have to say, and always refer to the manufacturer for proper instruction. The other important reason to refer to the manufacturer is that you would be surprised at the number of pool storeowners and builders who do not have a pool or a spa. It is hard to take advice from someone who has no personal knowledge and tries to give you advice.

Your warranty on your spa will also depend on how you maintain your spa and the water chemistry. Imbalanced water can scale and damage the heater, pumps, and other equipment. Upon filling the spa, it is very important to make sure that you bleed the system of any trapped air. How you should bleed the system will be described in the manual from the manufacturer.

Getting Your Spa in Working Condition

Assuming that you got the spa home and get the electrical properly connected, what should you do next? You must kill any bacteria, mildew, or mold that may be hiding in the spa.

Remove the filter(s), and if they are in good shape, soak them in a bucket with approximately 1 tablespoon of dichlor or 4 cups of liquid chlorine overnight. The next day, start filling up your spa. During this time, if the spa has come with a cover, make sure that it is clean and does not have any water trapped in it. If the cover is saturated, you can bet mold and other unwanted things are hidden in the cover and it needs to be replaced.

Once your spa is filled, go ahead and fill it to the top. Add 2 cups of dichlor or 1/2 gallon of liquid chlorine and turn it on. Let it run with the cover on, if you have one. Occasionally turn on the rest of the equipment and work the air valves to let the chlorine get into all the available lines and kill anything that you do not desire. Do not turn on the heater at this time.

Let the spa run for at least four hours to ensure all of the algae and bacteria are killed. Then go to your local pool and spa store and purchase an enzyme that will take out all the body oils and junk that is stuck inside your plumbing. After running this for an additional two hours — or whatever is recommended on the product that you use — it is time to drain your spa.

When you get it drained, take a water hose and wash all the jets thoroughly and let them drain. Keep circulating water through the jets until clear water is coming out of the drain of the spa. Once this is done, fill it back up to the proper level.

Going off the chart in Chapter 11, shock the spa again using dichlor or liquid chlorine and let it run for at least an hour. Leave the cover off to allow the chlorine to dissipate overnight.

The next day, check your chemical balance. If the chlorine level is below 5.0 ppm, check the rest of the chemistry and adjust it. It is a good idea to check the pH before you add the chlorine at both cleanings to ensure that the pH level is above 7.2.

Once your levels have been adjusted using the charts, you can turn on your heaters, close the cover, and let the spa do the job it is suppose to do. Start with a lower temperature like 95°F and see where it stabilizes. If the temperature is satisfactory, increase the temperature to 100°F. If it stops, it would appear that the thermostat and limit switches are working. To check this, make sure you use a good thermometer.

After the initial filling, when you open the cover, make sure that you do not breathe the mist that escapes into the atmosphere because it still may contain bacteria and mold spores that are not good for the lungs. If everything seems to work satisfactorily and you have adjusted the temperature to where you would like to start, it is time to climb in. Watch for irritation to your eyes. If you experience irritation after a couple of minutes, this is a good indication that your water may need more sanitation. If everything is okay, just follow the maintenance program included in this book and begin enjoying your spa.

As with a new spa, people tend to want to enjoy their used spa to the fullest. Start out slow, and increase your time and temperature gradually. It will take your body a few times to get used to being in hot water. If you experience trouble breathing or weak and tired muscles, it is time to get out.

Now that your spa is installed, and you are aware of the maintenance your spa and spa water will require, you should know the specific measurements for the chemicals you will be adding to your spa. This next chapter will detail the chemicals you will need to add to your water to keep it clean and safe for use.

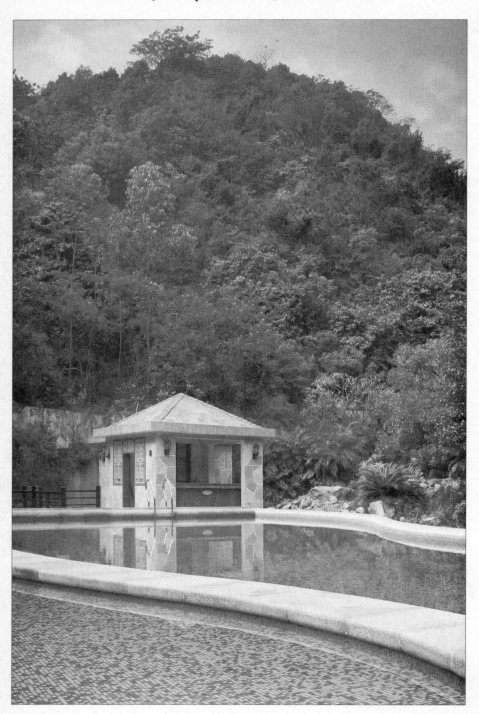

CHAPTER TEN

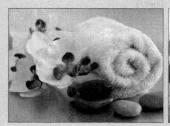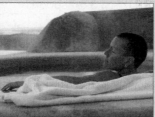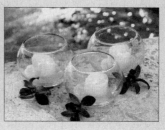

Chemical Treatment Charts

T here is a difference between liquid and dry measurements. Basic math skills are needed for calculations of spa water volume and chemical measurements. The best way to determine the volume of water in your spa is to consult your manufacturer. They know the volume, but it can differ depending on the level of water that is in the spa. It is always easier to add a little more than to take away any extra that is in the water. Before testing, make sure you run the spa for a couple of minutes to make sure everything is in solution to get an accurate test of the water.

Note: The first two charts below include approximate measurements. Liquid refers to fluid or volume, while dry refers to weight.

Liquid Measurements Conversion Chart			
1 teaspoon		$1/_3$ Tablespoon	5 milliliters
1 Tablespoon	½ ounce	3 teaspoons	15 milliliters
2 Tablespoons	1 ounce	$1/_8$ cup, 6 teaspoons	30 milliliters
¼ cup	2 fluid ounces	4 tablespoons	60 milliliters
½ cup	4 fluid ounces	8 tablespoons	118 milliliters
1 cup	8 fluid ounces	16 tablespoons	237 milliliters
2 cups	16 fluid ounces	1 pint	473 milliliters
1 pint	16 fluid ounces	½ quart	473 milliliters

Dry Measurements Conversion Chart		
1 ounce		28.35 (30) grams
4 ounces	¼ pound	125 grams
8 ounces	½ pound	240 grams
12 ounces	¾ pound	375 grams
16 ounces	1 pound	454 grams

Chemicals vary in strength depending on the manufacturer, and you should always read the label on the packaging for the percentage of active ingredient. Unfortunately, measurements for a spa make it more difficult to determine the right amount of chemical to apply, and sometimes it requires some guessing at measurements. The best that you can hope for is to be as accurate as you can and as careful as you can. Remember, not only are you dealing with a small volume of water, but also a very small dosage of chemicals.

This next chart has to deal with bromine. The best way to use this chart is to use sodium bromide and an equal part of potassium monopersulfate or dichlor. Note that the measurements for bromine give the dry measurement amount first and then the liquid measurement second.

Amount of Bromine to Raise 1 PPM	
250-400 gal (950-1512 liters)	2 grams-½ teaspoon
450-500 gal (1701-1870 liters)	3 grams-²/₃ teaspoon
1000 gal (3780 liters)	6 grams-1 teaspoon

When you look at the above chart, you might say there is no way to do an accurate measurement unless you have a small scale because it is almost impossible to get the measurement just right. These measurements have been rounded off to the closest measurement that you would have around your home. You should not really concern yourself so deeply with this. If you have a bromine bank established, the addition of a catalyst such as chlorine or potassium monopersulfate will reactivate the bromine that is in the bank. Using bromine tablets will maintain a good bromine level.

Most bromine tablets are put into a floating 1-inch tablet feeder, as are chlorine tablets. Active chemicals are released by eroding the tablet, causing the chemical to disperse in the water. The more chemical you want in the water, the lower you adjust the lower end of the feeder. They work very well as long as you keep the same amount of tablets in the feeder at all times to erode the same amount of chemical all the time. Bromine tablets usually weigh 18 grams. It is hard to calculate additional treatments for adjustments. All the brands of tablets have different bonding agents and dissolve in their own way. Once you get your chemicals the way you want them, stay with the same brand of chemicals.

Amount of Chlorine to Raise 1 PPM Chlorine Level			
% Available Chlorine	250 gallons 950 liters	400 gallons 1512 liters	1000 gallons 3780 liters
12.5 % (liquid)	¼ ounce	½ ounce	1.02 oz
65 %	1½ grams-⅓ tsp	2 ½ grams-½ tsp	1 ½ tsp
75 %	1 grams-⅓ tsp	½ tsp	1 tsp
90 %	¼ tsp	½ tsp	1 tsp

The measurements in the previous two charts are rounded off to the closest equivalent that you have the availability to measure. Because most people will not have the capability to measure such a small amount, they have been taken to the closest known measurement.

To lower pH, use either muriatic acid or sodium bisulfate. It is recommended that you use dry acid on a spa because it eliminates most chances of damaging the surface of the spa. Muriatic acid is cheaper to use, and a gallon could last you a year. You have to make the choice of price versus safety and protection of your spa.

These charts are a generic type. Because some spa owners will not use the liquid DPD test kits and may use the OTO or strips, these will get you in close range.

To Decrease pH Using Muriatic Acid

pH	250 Gallons 950 liters	400 Gallons 1512 liters	1000 Gallons 3780 liters
7.6 to 7.8	¼ ounce	½ ounce	1 ¼ ounces
7.8 to 8.0	¼ ounce	½ ounce	1 $\frac{1}{3}$ ounces
8.0 to 8.4	¼ ounce	½ ounce	1 ¼ ounces
Over 8.4	¾ ounce	1 ½ ounces	3 ounces

To Decrease pH Using Dry Acid

These dosages are estimated based on a certain chemical manufacturer and can differ from one manufacturer to another. Care must be used to establish the correct dosage.

PH	250 Gallons 950 liters	400 Gallons 1512 liters	1000 Gallons 3780 liters
7.6 to 7.8	¼ ounce	1 $\frac{1}{5}$ ounces	1 ½ ounces
7.8 to 8.0	$\frac{1}{3}$ ounce	$\frac{2}{3}$ ounce	1 ¾ ounces
8.0 to 8.4	$\frac{1}{5}$ ounce	1 $\frac{1}{5}$ ounces	3 ½ ounces
Over 8.4	¾ ounce	1 ½ ounces	5 ounces

To Lower Total Alkalinity Using Muriatic Acid

REDUCE BY	*SPA*	*VOLUME*	
PPM	250 Gallons 950 liters	400 Gallons 1512 liters	1000 Gallons 3780 liters
10	½ ounce liquid	1 ounce liquid	¼ cup liquid
20	1 ounce liquid	2 oz liquid	½ cup liquid
30	1 ½ ounces liquid	3 ounces liquid	6 ounces liquid
40	2 ounces liquid	4 ounces liquid	1 cup liquid
50	2 ½ ounces liquid	5 ounces liquid	1 $\frac{1}{3}$ cup liquid
60	3 ounces liquid	6 ounces liquid	1 ½ cup liquid
70	3 ½ ounces liquid	7 ounces liquid	1 $\frac{7}{8}$ cup liquid
81	4 ounces liquid	1 cup	2 cups-1 pint liquid
90	4 ½ ounces liquid	9 ounces liquid	1 ¼ pts liquid

To Lower Total Alkalinity Using Dry Acid			
Dry acid is safer to use than muriatic acid and should be dissolved in water before adding to spa.			
REDUCE BY	SPA	VOLUME	
PPM	250 Gallons 950 liters	400 Gallons 1512 liters	1000 Gallons 3780 liters
10	1 tablespoon or ½ ounce	1 ounce	2 ½ ounces
20	2 tablespoons or 1 ounce	2 ounces	$^2/_3$ cup
30	¼ cup	2 ½ ounces	1 cup
40	2 ½ ounces	4 ounces	1 ¼ cup
50	3 ounces	5 ounces	1 ½ cup
60	½ cup	6 ounces	2 cups
70	¾ cup	1 cup	2 ¼ cups
81	¾ cup	1 cup and 1 ounce	2 ½ cups
90	$^7/_8$ cup	1 $^1/_3$ cups	3 cups

To Raise pH Using Soda Ash

In a spa with a very small volume of water, plain soda ash is a very difficult product to add because the proper amounts to add are so small. If you are adjusting total alkalinity using sodium bicarbonate, it has a pH of only 8.2, which is all that it will raise the pH.

The chart below was developed in accordance with Taylor's DPD test kit. Apply your own adjustments as you see fit. The volumes of water listed are 400 and 1,000 gallons. If you have a smaller or larger spa, then you have to add less or more for your volume level depending on your source water and the sanitizer that you are using. Increasing the pH is usually required when too much acid has been added and corrections have to be made. This is not always the case, though.

Always adjust the total alkalinity first over the pH adjustment. Because sodium bicarbonate has a pH of 8.2, trying to lower the pH and then raise alkalinity is useless. Adjust your total akalinity, then test and adjust pH if necessary the next day.

Drops of reagent	400 gallons – 1512 liters	1000 gallons – 3780 liters
1 drop	0.2 ounce	0.5 ounce
2 drops	0.4 ounce	1.02 ounces
3 drops	0.6 ounce	1.5 ounces
4 drops	0.8 ounce	2.0 ounces
5 drops	1.0 ounce	2.5 ounces

To Increase Alkalinity Using Baking Soda (Sodium Bicarbonate, 100 Percent)			
Desired increase in ppm	250 Gallons 950 liters	400 Gallons 1512 liters	1000 Gallons 3780 liters
10	.5 ounce	.9 ounce	2.25 ounce
20	1.0 ounce	1.8 ounce	4.5 ounces
30	1.5 ounces	2.7 ounces	6.75 ounces
40	2.0 ounces	3.6 ounces	9.0 ounces
50	2.25 ounces	4.5 ounces	11.25 ounces

Super-Chlorination (Shocking)

If you are using chlorine as a sanitizer, you may find that you experience a strong odor of chlorine. This is referred to as chloramines. The chlorine is locked up with ammonia and/

or nitrogen and other things in the water and they combine together. This means the chlorine is not free and has limited effects as an oxidizer. The term **breakpoint chlorination** refers to the addition of more chlorine to break up the chloramines and restore the sanitizing ability of the free chlorine.

The bromamines are different because they still have a sanitizing ability and do not need to be broken up. Just by keeping the daily levels up to at least 2 ppm without an ozonator and 1 ppm using an ozonator, you should be okay for a portable spa.

To shock a spa, you need about a 30 ppm level of chlorine and should hold for about four hours. The following chart shows the 30 ppm shock table for algae removal which will work well for shocking your spa. To simplify things, it is easier to use PM after every use — that generally will keep everything in line.

Shock Table (30 PPM)			
% of available chlorine	250 Gallons 950 liters	400 Gallons 1512 liters	1000 Gallons 3780 liters
12.5 (liquid)	8 ounces	12.8 ounces	32 ounces (1 quart)
65	1.5 ounce	2.5 ounces	6.2 ounces
75	1.4 ounces	2.25 ounces	5.6 ounces
90	1 ounce	1.6 ounces	4 ounces

It is extremely important to read the label of your product to determine the percentage of available chlorine to get your dosages correct.

Algae Removal

There is really no reason for a covered spa to ever get algae if it is maintained properly. On occasions, an uncovered spa may get a case of algae from exposure to the elements. In any case, if you get algae, brush the spa down well in all the affected areas and around the jets and features, then follow the chart above and let the spa run for at least four hours. Turn the heat off, let it run, and filter. It is important to run as many features as you can to make sure the sanitizer flows to all the areas of the spa to kill the algae that is hiding in the piping and other plumbing features. If you notice that the flow starts to slow down, remove the filter, clean it well, and continue. If you have black or mustard-colored algae, then add equal amounts of sodium bromide with the chlorine to help eliminate the algae.

After the algae are dead, drain the spa. Once drained, you need to flush out the jets and features with water, clean the filter, and make sure there are no signs of algae before filling.

The next chapter will take you from the maintenance of a standard spa to the accommodations you will need to make for a specialty spa.

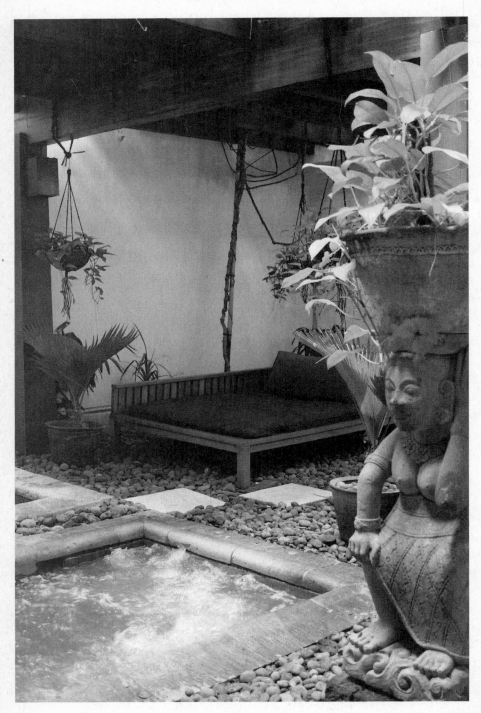

CHAPTER ELEVEN

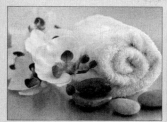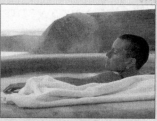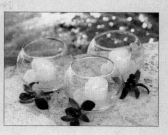

Specialty Tubs and Spas

There are specialty spas, as they are called, that are designed for a special purpose. Some are more like small pools, but they are designed for therapy and exercise. These vary in design depending on the manufacturer. As with all pool products, there are different manufacturers for these tubs and spas and different versions and models available. Some feature a one-piece shell, and others are installed and lined with vinyl. The vinyl-lined spas are designed for places where there is no room to move the whole tub, such as a basement.

The original swim spas were designed to allow you to get exercise and swim without going anywhere. What that means is they incorporate a high volume flow of water that lets you swim in one spot, much like a treadmill allows you to run without traveling anywhere. It is like swimming against a current in the ocean or against waves. The flow of water can be adjusted depending on your ability to swim. This allows professional Olympic swimmers to train at their homes without having to go to a pool every day. It also allows you a great source of exercise and prevents you from having to create enough room on your property to accommodate a large swimming pool.

Some of these have large volume pumps, and some actually have paddles that flow the water. Some are made in one piece, and others come in many pieces so you can install them in a room in your home, basement, or garage. The popularity of these spas is growing significantly. These spas are usually heated and can be used for exercise and many types of therapy. They also hold many people because they are larger than a typical spa.

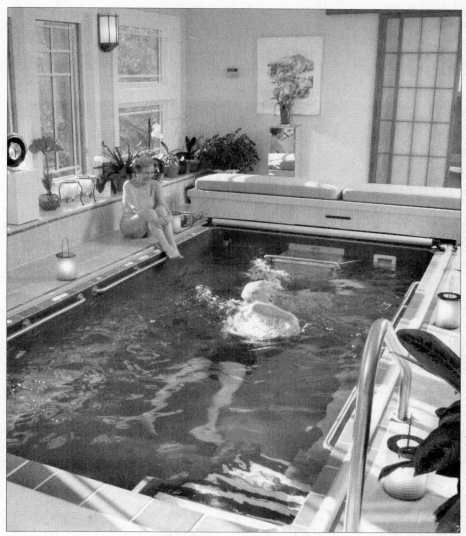

Figure 11-1 is a swim spa from Endless Pools® that was installed indoors. Courtesy of Endless Pools

Another example is below. With the small size of the pool, it is easy to put it almost anywhere and makes it perfect to use in the privacy of your home. This type of pool is great for massage therapy and water exercises.

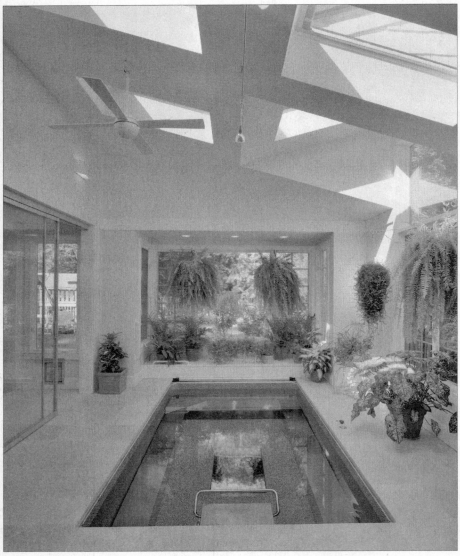

Figure 11-2 is the Ridgeway model by Endless Pools®, which is also installed indoors. Courtesy of Endless Pools

For people who have health problems, exercise and therapy can be critical to their health. This type of product helps ensure a person receives proper exercise and therapy in the comfort of his or her home. Having your therapy in your home eliminates the feeling of embarrassment that some have working out in a public facility. Using a pool for swimming is also one of the best exercises that you can do.

Endless Pools® does something that most companies do not: they have a Test Swim Program where you can arrange to actually try out a pool in your area or travel to a factory showroom for a trial use. It would be well worth a trip to be able to make a decision on a product when you know what it can do for you.

Wooden Hot Tubs

Before acrylic and other composite spas were used, the original spas were wooden hot tubs. Some were made out of redwood, red cedar, Alaskan yellow cedar, and teak as well as some artificial composite construction. These tubs are heated in a variety of ways. You have the regular gas and electric versions as well as wood-fired tubs.

These hot tubs offer a traditional and unique look. The look of beautiful wood is more pleasing than a manicured piece of acrylic, though the functional characteristics of a wooden hot tub are not nearly as therapeutic as an acrylic spa that is designed for therapy.

If you are interested in building a wooden spa, it is not that difficult. But as with most things, buying it already made has fewer frustrations. The service and warranty issue is a very big consideration when you decide to build your own spa. If you want to build your own wooden hot tub, it is recommended that you buy a kit from a manufacturer that includes the equipment and put it together yourself on location. In the long run, it will not cost you very much more to have the manufacturer build and ship the tub, and there will be fewer headaches than if you decide to put the spa together yourself.

One such company that makes hot tub kits is SeaOtter Wood-Works, Inc. The company is located in Haines, Alaska, and not only has their own models but will also custom build you a hot tub. Products that are built in Alaska are capable of enduring the harsh temperatures and other related weather problems, which makes for a good product.

If you want to reduce stress and are looking for basic and relaxing therapy, you may consider looking into this company or others like it. The main concern with a wooden hot tub is that it has to be maintained properly. Wood absorbs water, which contains bacteria. If not properly maintained, wooden tubs can be more of a problem than a spa made out of acrylic or other products.

If you want to do something special to a hot tub, contact the manufacturer and ask them if they will incorporate a set of jets or other things into the hot tub. Custom-made hot tubs can be designed with your own variations. It all comes down to the money you are willing to spend.

Heating systems vary on the different hot tubs. Some have solar heat to help heat the water. Some systems use electric heat, gas, or wood. The differences are strictly a matter of preference. With wood heat you need to monitor the tem-perature more closely, but it will cost you less if you have access to large quantities of hardwood. Wood heat requires you to do more labor but at a reduced cost in expenses.

In the northern states of the United States, wood heat is used to heat pools. The wood heaters cost, on average, less than a gas heater or heat pump. The advantage to the wood heater is that after the initial expense, the cost is only what you have to pay to supply firewood. Like solar heating, the expense of heating is very small compared to the alternatives.

Interior Whirlpool Tubs

An interior whirlpool tub is an item most people have seen when viewing a new home. It is a bathtub that has jets that circulate the water for massage in the comfort of your private bath. It uses the hot water from your hot water heater and has a circulation pump for water flow. However, these tubs have no filtration. As was stated earlier, the filter is the heart of a spa or pool. The idea behind this is that when you are done using the water, you just simply drain it and start with new water the next time. How wrong this assumption is.

When you look inside these tubs, you will see what looks like an average spa with a suction port and return jets. The tub will have a pump but no filtration, which is where the problem arises. When you are finished, you drain the water out of the tub. What you do not do is drain the water out of the pump and the lines. Usually, there is quite a bit of water left in the system that just sits there growing bacteria. When you fill up the tub, whether you turn on the system or not, bacteria and other unwanted things will enter the water that a bather is using. Soaps, lotions, and other paraphernalia that has washed off the bather also get trapped in the lines and equipment when the tub is emptied. Because of the trapped water, it is truly not a healthy environment to be in.

If you own one of these types of tubs, it is recommended that you use some PM in it regularly before draining. If you have a spa tub and you bathe young children in it, do not fill the tub above the intake or returns. This will keep the old water trapped and separated from the water the children are sitting in. The young and old are less tolerant to bacteria and disease than most of us.

Now that you have learned about the various types of specialty tubs available on the market and the pros and cons of each, you need to know the steps to take to properly maintain your spa. This next chapter will walk you through the directions to keep your spa running efficiently.

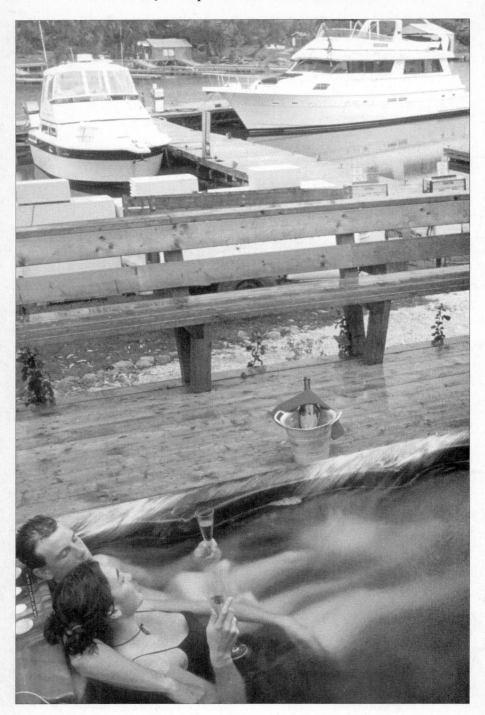

CHAPTER TWELVE

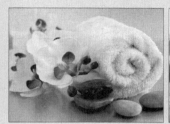 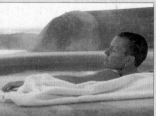 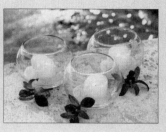

Step-by-Step Maintenance

B ecause every spa will be different due to the bather load, how often it is used, the source water, and the sanitizer being used, it is only possible to provide you with the basic guidelines and general rules of spa maintenance. As with a pool, each spa will be different, which in turn will make its maintenance schedule different. This chapter will provide you with a happy medium.

To start, assume that the spa is set up and is running. When you get ready to use your spa, you should first open the cover and let the mist clear. While this is happening, it is a perfect time to shower before entering the spa. Depending on your ventilation, a couple of minutes to clear the air should be enough. Check your water temperature and adjust it if you are one that turns the temperature down after use. The next thing is to test the water. What you are looking for is the level of sanitizer and if the pH is too high or low. Also, you want to make sure that the water inside the spa is at the correct level so the pumps can function properly and not damage any equipment. If the spa is low on water and air is getting into the suction side, it can cause air bubbles. When the water goes into the heater and it has air in the line, it can damage the heating element or cause the heater to operate improperly.

If you need to add water or adjust the sanitizer or pH, you can do it now and wait for half an hour and retest before entry. If everything is acceptable and you had your session in your spa, it is recommended that you add a couple of ounces of PM and let the spa run for 15 more minutes before you shut it down. This will help break up the ammonia by-products that will be left in the water from the perspiration, oils, and contaminates off your body. It is also advisable for you to take another shower to remove the sanitizer that is on your skin so your body does not absorb it through your skin.

For a regular maintenance schedule, it is recommended that you test your water twice a week. Do not go longer than once a week without testing your spa. Improper water balance can scale quickly in warm water, and if the water is acidic then it can damage equipment fairly rapidly.

To perform regular maintenance, the first thing to do is to open your spa cover and let the mist blow in the wind. If you see particles of debris in the bottom of the spa or on the seats, use your spa vacuum to remove the unwanted material. Turn the pumps on to let the water circulate properly and mix up the water well. Let it run for at least ten minutes; then you can reach in the center of the spa — away from a water return — and collect a sample for testing. Test your sample and adjust your water. While your spa is running and mixing the chemicals you added, it is a good time to take a sponge and wipe down the surface that is out of the water, especially the water line area, to remove the oils and lotions that have deposited on the walls of your spa. Use a clean sponge that has no soap or other chemicals on it. Make sure that you clean the area of the cover that seals the surface of the spa and cover as well as the entire underneath of the cover. If you have a skimmer, then clean it as well if you can at this time.

Once the spa has run for half an hour, retest your water if you made adjustments to it. If everything is okay, remove your filters and clean them well. If you soak them in a cleaning solution, make sure that you rinse them well because you do not want any detergents left on the filters. If you have hard water or have a good deal of iron in your water, you may want to acid wash the filters after you clean them. If you have iron on your filters, you can simply soak them in a bucket with citric acid for 15 minutes and then rinse them off. Citric acid will remove the iron from your cartridge filters. After rinsing them well, re-install them. Once you install them back in the spa, turn the spa on, check for air locks, and make sure that the pumps circulate well without any flow interruptions or strange noises from the pump. After you have your spa for a while, you will be able to tell from just the noise whether something is wrong. A good visible inspection before you start checking your spa will tell you if you have any leaks.

That is about all you have to do to maintain your spa. Some other things for you to look for are excessive foaming when you turn on your spa, smelly water, discolored water, or a gritty feeling on your surface. If you experience this, drain your spa with the cleaning procedures detailed in the previous chapters, because this could be an indication that you are leaving the water in too long. If this happens, start replacing the water more frequently. Draining will not cure all of your problems if you do not clean the water properly. Once a proper cleaning is done, refill your spa and start over. Make sure that you check for air locks in the system according to the manufacturer's recommendations.

Something else for you to consider is to clean the location where the spa is located. A tub of water is a magnet for things that float in the air. If the area is dirty, there are good chances that walking on the dirty area will contaminate the water. Debris that blows in the air will also find its way in the spa. As the normal dust goes over the top of the spa and makes contact with the mist coming off the surface of the water, the combination of dirt and vapor makes the particles too heavy to float, and they will fall in the water. Keeping a clean area will be beneficial to maintain the spa.

If you bought a used spa and you do not have the manufacturer's recommendations for maintaining your spa, go online and download them. You may have other equipment that needs to be checked periodically. You will quickly learn what should be running. An ozonator will run whenever the pumps are on. The heater will work when the thermostat senses the temperature is too low. The pumps should come on without delay when commanded to.

Always test all of your equipment. Even a simple thing like a light out could mean that a leak has corroded something. If something does not work, get it repaired immediately, especially if the item is part of the circulation equipment. A pump that is not needed for the functions you want to use means water is sitting in a pipe somewhere gathering bacteria because it is not being circulated and filtered. If you have a spa with only 400 gallons of water in it, then it does not take much debris to contaminate the water.

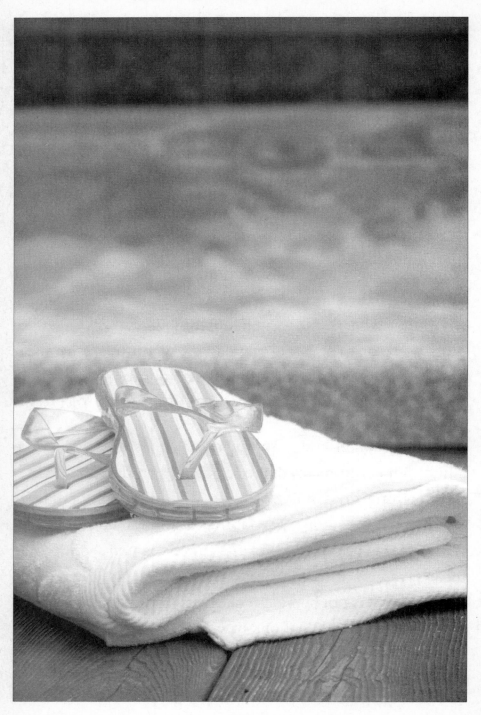

CONCLUSION

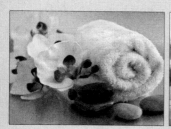 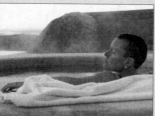 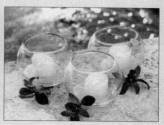

After finishing reading this book, you now have all the knowledge you will need to properly care for your hot tub or spa. Owning a spa can be a highly enjoyable experience, but if you do not maintain your spa, you can risk exposing yourself to disease or suffering an adverse reaction from improper water maintenance. By following the information in this guide, you will ensure that your time as a spa owner is an enjoyable and healthy experience.

Happy soaking!

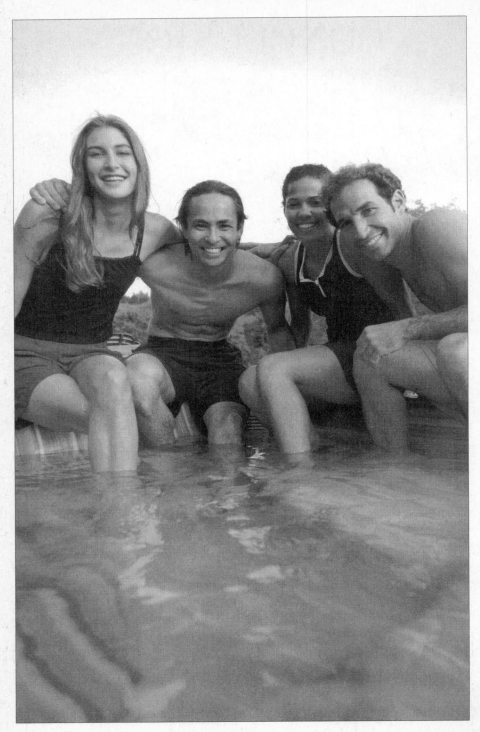

GLOSSARY OF TERMS

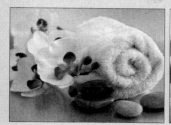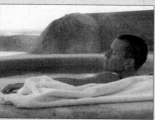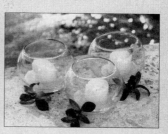

ACID: An acid, whether liquid or dry, has the ability to lower pH and alkalinity in water. Also, muriatic acid can be used to acid wash a pool and remove unwanted stains and scale from pool surfaces.

ACID DEMAND: A test that determines the amount of acid that is required to lower the pH in water.

ACID RAIN: Rain having an unusually low pH, usually 4.5 or lower, which is caused by pollutants in the atmosphere.

ACID WASH: Acid wash describes using a mixture of muriatic acid and water at different ratios to clean the plaster on your pool surface.

ACRYLIC: A material that is usually formed by heat and a mold, using vacuum to form an object. Portable spas are made of acrylic.

AERATOR: A vented pipe installed in the plumbing, mainly in spas, that can have an adjustment of air that is introduced into a water line before returning to the body of water.

AIR BLOWER: A fan-type motor that forces air into a spa to agitate the water.

AIR BUTTON: A device used to control blowers, lights, and jet pumps.

AIR CONTROL: A device that controls the amount of air that can go to certain types of jets or functions to make them more or less aggressive.

AIR LOCKS: These are cause when air is trapped inside spa lines and equipment.

AIR RELIEF VALVE: A valve that is located on a spa or pool filter that allows you to remove the air that is trapped so that it does not cloud the water.

AIR SWITCH: This feature is mostly on spas and in-home whirlpool baths and allows you to turn the pump on by pushing an air button that activates a switch in another location. This turns on equipment such as pumps and blowers. These come in single or multiple functions.

ALGAE: A microscopic living plant or plant-like organism with more than 21,000 different varieties. Normal pool algae are green, yellow, or black, with an additional form of algae that is called pink and is not a real algae but a fungus. These organisms usually grow in water or on surfaces and can become airborne to contaminate other water sources. Some are chlorine resistant and are hard to kill.

ALGAECIDE: Algaecides are designed to kill algae and aid in the prevention of reoccurrences of algae.

ALGAESTAT: An algaestat retards and prevents growth of algae. Some algaecides are only algaestats and should be looked at carefully.

ALGAE SPORES: A dormant form of algae residing in atmospheric conditions. They are introduced into the pool or spa by rain, winds, and dust storms.

ALKALINE: When water has a pH higher than 7.0.

ALKALINITY: Alkalinity refers to the water in an above acidic state, or above a pH of 7.0. It acts as a buffer for pH and aids in controlling the correct pH in normal recommended parameters. Alkalinity also aids in the prevention of spiking in pH levels.

ALUMINUM SULFATE: Sometimes called a clarifier; the main ingredient alum gathers smaller particles together and makes larger particles. These particles are dropped to the bottom of the pool and are usually removed with a vacuum so that they do not re-enter the pool. Also know as flocculants, they are mainly used as a last resort to clear cloudy water and to remove unwanted particles in water.

AMBIENT TEMPERATURE: The temperature of the surrounding atmosphere.

ANSI: American National Standards Institute. This organization sets construction standards.

APHA: American Public Health Association. This is a national public health and safety organization.

AMMONIA: Very soluble combination of nitrogen and hydrogen (NH3) that when introduced in pool water at certain levels can tie up free chlorine levels to make chloramines. In bromine pools and spas, it makes bromamines that makes the sanitizers weak and ineffective.

AMPERAGE (AMPS): The measurement of electricity that equals watts divided by voltage.

ANTISIPHON VALVE: A valve designed to stop the flow of water going back to a certain source.

ANTISURGE VALVE: A check valve that is used in pool and spa plumbing to prevent water from entering the blower assembly.

ANTIVORTEX: Commonly used in the description of a main drain cover in a pool or spa to limit the whirlpool effect when water is pulled through it.

AROMATHERAPY: A form of therapy that uses special scents.

ASCORBIC ACID: A compound that removes iron stains from vinyl liners and fiberglass pools and spas.

AVAILABLE CHLORINE: Free chlorine that is readily available to sanitize the water and is not locked up with ammonia.

BACKWASH: The reversal of water in filters to remove unwanted particles and clean the filter so that flow is established to a proper level for the removal of contaminants.

BACTERIA: Microorganisms that may be introduced in pool or spa water and can be dangerous to the health of humans.

BALANCED WATER: When the chemical parameters are at the appropriate levels and are in balance with each other: total alkalinity, pH, calcium hardness, and temperature. As measured using the Langelier Index, these should equal zero.

BALL VALVE: A valve that has a ball in the center with a sized hole through it so that flow can be controlled.

BASE: An alkaline chemical that will counteract the pH of an acid.

BASE DEMAND: A test used to figure out the proper amount of base needed to raise the pH of pool or spa water, which could be soda ash (sodium carbonate) or sodium bicarbonate if alkalinity needs to be raised.

BIGUANIDES: Sanitizers that use the polymer PHMB, a non-halogen sanitizer for pool and spa use. However, this peroxide-based chemical cannot kill algae alone.

BLOWER: A device that blows air through piping to give spa jets a bubbling effect.

BOBBIE: A sock that attaches to a hose that acts as a filter for metals and other contaminants.

BONDING: The process of connecting the pool shell reinforcement rod, the light, and all metal construction materials to prevent electrolysis. All tie together and are grounded by a rod inserted in the ground.

BREAKPOINT CHLORINATION: Also called shocking. This is adding an amount of chlorine to a chlorinated pool to destroy chloramines, which is a combination of chlorine and ammonia that comes from bathers' sweat and urine. Chloramines tie up free available chlorine that is ineffective as a sanitizer. A recommended dose of 30 to 50 ppm will not only destroy chloramines but also kill most algae.

BROADCASTING: Dispensing chemicals by throwing them over the vast portion of the surface of the water.

BROMAMINES: Combined bromine and ammonia with the ability to sanitize, unlike chloramines.

BROMINE: A member of the halogen family often used as a spa sanitizer because it is resistant to hot water. This is not commonly used in pools because of its cost and is unstable and highly aggressive if water balance is not kept within parameters.

BROMINE BANK: This occurs when inactive bromine ions group together in a mass that can be reactivated when chlorine is added.

BTU: Stands for British Thermal Unit; the amount of heat required to increase 1 pound of water 1°F in temperature.

BUFFER: A base such as sodium bicarbonate that resists sudden changes in pH called spiking.

BYPASS: An arrangement of valves that are designed to redirect the flow of water to a piece of equipment. They are also used to control flow to a certain equipment part or device.

CALCIUM: A metal ion contained in water that is able to form salts such as calcium carbonate, causing cloudiness and/or scaling. This can be caused by an imbalance of pH.

CALCIUM BLEED: For pools, it is when the calcium leaches from the plaster. This is normal on new surfaces but can be extreme if balance is not correct.

CALCIUM CARBONATE: Scale. This is a major component that is precipitated from the water and becomes attached to pool surfaces and in equipment and piping. Levels can rise due to the addition of calcium in many forms. Salt pools have a higher TDS of calcium as well as hard water sources. The use of calcium hypochlorite also adds to this level of hardness.

CALCIUM CHLORIDE: A salt that is used to increase levels of calcium hardness in pool and spa water.

CALCIUM HARDNESS: The level of the mineral calcium dissolved in the pool water.

CALCIUM HYPOCHLORITE: Commonly called cal hypo or HTH. This is a granular form of chlorine that comes in different strengths of total chlorine. This adds to TDS but is fairly safe to use; however, it is an unstable form of chlorine. It cannot be mixed with any other chemical due to danger of chemical explosion. Addition of acid to this element will result in chlorine gas, which can be lethal.

CARBON DIOXIDE: A gas that, when it is present in the water, usually feeds algae for growth and is introduced in several forms. Algae thrive on carbon dioxide.

CAUSTIC: Capable of eating or destroying by chemical action.

CAVITATION: When the discharge of the pump either exceeds the suction of the pump or a restriction causes the vacuum to collapse from the impeller of the pump. This can be caused by a clogged impeller.

CHITIN: A tough, semitransparent polymer found in the shells of crabs and lobsters. Chitin is contained in the product SeaKlear and serves as a coagulant for oils, metals, and organic materials. It makes the small particles combine together to make larger particles that can be taken out by the filter.

CHELATOR: A water-soluble molecule that is able to bond with metal ions, which keeps them from coming out of suspension and staining and/or scaling pool or spa surfaces and equipment. It keeps metals in solution so the filter can remove them.

CHECK VALVE: A device that lets water flow in one direction and not in the other direction.

CHLORAMINES: The combination of chlorine and ammonia or nitrogen that when it is combined creates an unwanted odor and limits the sanitizing ability of chlorine.

CHLORINE: A member of the halogen family of sanitizers. It is available in liquid, gas, or granular forms in different strengths. Some are stabilized and some are unstable.

CHLORINE DEMAND: Amount of free available chlorine that the water needs or demands to raise the residue of chlorine to a certain level.

CHLORINE LOCK: This applies to chloramines that have no ability to sanitize properly and need to be shocked to release the chlorine in a free state. This is also called breakpoint chlorination.

CHLORINE NEUTRALIZER: A chemical that makes chlorine useless or neutral.

CIRCULATION PUMP: In relation to pools, this is the pump that circulates water for a particular purpose in the system.

CLARIFIER: A clarifier is a product that attracts small particles in the water so they become larger particles, allowing the filter to remove them.

CONDUCTION: When energy flows from an area of higher temperatures to an area of lower temperatures.

CONTAMINANTS: Described as making water unfit for use because of the introduction of unwholesome or undesirable elements that can cause cloudiness of the water.

CONTROL PANEL: A pad mounted on the spa that allows you to turn on different devices.

CONVECTION: When energy is transferred into or out of an object by the movement of the surrounding water.

CONVERSION: When one form of energy transforms into another form.

COPING: The top part of the pool that ties the pool and the deck together. This usually has an overhang and can be made of brick, concrete, pavers, wood, or plastic.

COPPER: An element that is used in many pool products as an algaecide. It can stain surfaces if not properly used.

COPPER SULFATE: Nicknamed bluestone; a granular substance that is used to kill algae and also has a flocking ability.

CONDITIONER: Commonly called stabilizer. Usually cyanuric acid, it slows the decomposition of chlorine products.

CORROSION: Wearing away of metal objects gradually in degrees, usually as the result of a chemical reaction caused by imbalanced water that dissolves metals or minerals.

CORROSION RESISTANT: The ability to maintain original surface characteristics under prolonged use.

CYANURIC ACID: Stabilizes pool water so the residue of chlorine is not affected as much by the sun. This element is not needed in indoor pools and should not be used with bromine products.

CYCLE: The completion of running the pool pump by turning over all the water in the pool in 8 to 10 hours. From start to stop is one cycle. In a spa, it usually takes 30 minutes to turn over all the water in the pool.

DEAD ZONE: An area in the pool that has poor or no circulation that allows particles to cling to the wall and floor. These areas will usually be the first to get a bloom of algae.

DECK: The area that surrounds the pool. It can be made of many materials.

DEFOAMER: A product that is designed to remove the foam on the surface of the water in a spa.

DELAMINATING: When the acrylic and backing separates from the spa and bubbles appear on the surface.

DIATOMACEOUS EARTH (DE): A light, friable, siliceous material derived mainly from diatoms, or colonial algae. The white powder used in DE filters as a filter media filters out very small particles.

DICHLOR: Sodium dichloro-s-triazinetrione. A soluble form of chlorine that easily dissolves and is stabilized. It is an excellent sanitizer, but the cost makes it unpopular. It dissolves quickly, does not cloud the water, and has a long shelf life. It is the second most expensive chlorine on the market. Care should be taken when shocking a pool with dichlor because of the addition of stabilizer that is mixed in with the chlorine. It has a pH close to 7.0, which is neutral.

DIFFUSER: A component inside a pool circulation pump that actually slows down the flow of water to make it more stable and increase pressure. It covers the impeller and has slots, holes, or veins that precisely control the flow of water.

DPD: Diethy-phenylene diamene. DPD testing allows you to determine total and free available chlorine levels in pool or spa water.

DRY ACID: Sodium bisulfate; a granular form of acid. It is mostly used in spas or with elderly pool and spa owners. This element is safer to use and distribute.

EFFECTIVE FILTRATION AREA: The total surface of a medium, which the designed flow rate will maintain during filtration.

ELECTROLYSIS: Two or more dissimilar metals passing through water with an electrical current. This causes light rings to turn black and can stain surfaces.

ELEMENT: The actual filter inside the filter body that traps the small particles of unwanted debris in water.

ENZYMES: Complex proteins that cause specific chemical changes in other substances without being affected themselves. This product is used in pools and spas to remove scum, odors, and the ring around the water line that consists of oils, makeup, and by-products that contaminate pool water and make it cloudy. They are also good for cleaning filter elements. Most dishwashing liquids have enzymes in them to dissolve these by-products.

EPA: The abbreviation for the Environmental Protection Agency.

FIBER OPTICS: A light used in pools and spas that has a source that is not near the water and lends the light down the fiber-optic cable that illuminates wherever it is exposed.

FILTER: A piece of equipment — the most important part of a pool and spa system — that is designed to remove unwanted particles in the water. Filters vary in the size of particles that they can remove.

FINGER FILTER: A new form of filter that has long, narrow "fingers" that the water passes through.

FIRE UP: A term used by the pool industry that starts the treatment of water on a new pool or one that has been drained. It usually consists of basic water chemistry, shocking the new water to kill bacteria, and regulating the levels of chemistry to protect a new surface during curing.

FOAMING: When soaps, oils, and other by-products make thick bubbles over the surface of the pool or spa water. This happens mostly in spas with a small volume of water. Some algaecides and algaestats create foaming.

FLOCCULANT: A product that acts as a clarifier by attracting the smaller particles and combining them in larger particles that drop to the bottom of the pool to allow you to vacuum them.

FLOW RATE: The volume of water, measured in gallons, that describes the amount of water passing through an object.

FREE CHLORINE: The available chlorine residue not tied up with any other element that is available for sanitizing water. This is the level that remains after the demand is satisfied.

GPM: Gallons per minute. This is a unit that measures the amount of liquid that flows in one minute.

GROUND FAULT CIRCUIT INTERPRETER: Commonly called a GFCI. This unit protects high voltage and low voltage on your control box.

GROUND FAULT INTERRUPTER: Commonly called a GFI. This is a device that is designed to interrupt the electrical flow to help prevent electrocution.

HALOGEN: The family of elements such as bromine, chlorine, fluorine, and iodine that are considered oxidizing agents or sanitizers.

HAMMERHEAD: A piece of equipment for vacuuming a pool that has an electric motor in it to pull debris from the bottom of the pool and up into a containment bag.

HARD WATER: The term of a high calcium level in pool and spa water caused by calcium and magnesium.

HARDWIRING: Using a directly wired cable from the spa to the electrical source that does not use plugs and connectors, making it a permanent connection.

HEATER: A piece of equipment used on spas and pools that raises the temperature of water to a desired limit. Pool heaters can be wood-fired, electric, oil, and gas-powered units.

HEAT EXCHANGER: The part of the heater that absorbs the heat and distributes it to the water to raise the temperature of the water in a pool or spa.

HEAT PUMP: A piece of equipment that removes the heat from the air and transfers it to pool water.

HORSEPOWER: Ratings of pool motors and equipment. It takes 746 watts of electricity to make 1 hp. One hp is the power it would take to raise 550 pounds to 1 foot in one second of time.

HYDRATION: A product of adding some type of moisture to a dry substance that combines to become one product.

HYDROTHERAPY: A form of treatment that uses water either internally or externally to treat medical conditions.

IMPELLER: A part of a centrifugal pump connected to the shaft of the armature in an electric motor that rotates at a set speed, usually 3600 rpm. It flows water and creates suction in the intake line, drawing water to the pump.

IMPURITIES: Substances dissolved or suspended in water that alters its chemical and physical properties.

INTERFERENCE: When two elements do not work well together.

IODINE: A sanitizer for water that is not commonly used in pools. It is a member of the halogen family and is commonly used in the purification of drinking water. It kills bacteria and prevents algae growth. It can stain surfaces.

IONIZER: A device that is either in a light form or injection. The injection is usually created by dissolving metal such as copper by an electrical charge and dissolving it in pool water. An ionizer works as an electric algaecide.

IRON: Iron is usually introduced into a pool or spa by either the source water or by something that is metal that has been in contact with the water. Chemicals can be used to keep the iron in solution and remove them from surfaces and let the filter take them out. Iron can be seen on the returns and main drain covers first and should be treated. Letting metals go without treatment can stain the surface of the pool, and you may not be able to get all of the stains out even with acid washing.

LANGELIER INDEX: The Langelier Saturation Index is a means of evaluating the water quality information to determine if the water is corrosive or scale forming. Even with water being close to the zero rating — neutral or balanced water — corrosion can still occur.

LATERALS: The tubes in the bottom of a sand filter that take in the filtered water for the return to the pool. During a backwash, the water is reversed and comes through the laterals, forcing water up through the sand to wash the particles from the sand to the waste port to be removed from the filter.

LEAF EATER: A cleaning tool that hooks up to a water hose and has a small micron bag to collect debris in a pool. The water is shot through small holes in the opening of the cleaner, shooting water up at an angle and causing suction. This sucks debris into the bag to be removed from the pool. This system works great on leaves. There are two models: one has wheels for concrete pools, and the other has a brush that goes around the bottom of the cleaner for vinyl pools.

LEAF RAKE: A large net that hooks to a pool pole that is used to skim the surface of a pool or remove debris from the bottom of the pool. Different sizes are available to remove either standard debris or fine micron nets to remove small debris.

LIMIT SWITCHES: Sensors that determine the temperature of the water.

LITHIUM HYPOCHLORITE: Chemical formula $LIOCl$; produced by bubbling chlorine gas through a solution of lithium, sodium, and potassium sulfate. This can be used directly on vinyl pools. It dissolves rapidly and is an unstable form of chlorine that requires stabilizer. It is the most expensive of the halogen family.

MAGNESIUM: A mineral found in water that contributes to water hardness and turbidity.

MAIN DRAIN: The drain or multiple drains in the bottom of a pool, or the side of a fiberglass pool or spa, that is an intake for the water in the lower section of the water. Without a main drain, the lower section of a deep pool can become a dead zone, which would be a perfect breeding ground for algae.

MANIFOLD: This is usually the same size as the internal water dimensions of the water line or it is larger. It has multiple connections for the water lines to go to different jets or sets of jets.

MARCITE: A product that is used as a plaster for the surface of a pool. Most marcite products contain no marble aggregates.

MEDIA: A substance that is used primarily in a DE filter to act as the filtering component that gathers small debris. When it is saturated, it can be backwashed out of the filter for the addition of new media.

METAL IONIZATION SYSTEM: Commonly known as ionizers; they have an electronic charge that produces metal ions from copper, silver, or both that kills bacteria and algae when disbursed in the water.

MISSION CLAMP: A device where the inner section is rubber and the outer section is usually stainless steel. Clamps surround the stainless steel portion to be tightened up to secure a watertight connection in a repair. It can be used on different kinds of pipes.

MICRON: A measurement that equals 1 millionth of a meter.

MICROORGANISM: A living, breathing creature. This is the reason a sanitizer has to be used in pool and spa water.

MULTI-PORT VALVE: This device allows the spa owner to filter; backwash; allow the water to bypass the filter and go out the discharge port to waste; and allow the water to circulate without going through the filter.

MURIATIC ACID: The liquid form of hydrochloric acid used to lower pH and alkalinity in pool or spa water. It can be used as a cleaning agent for concrete, bricks, scale, and irons and can also be used to remove the calcium and metal buildup on cartridge and DE filters.

NEGATIVE EDGE: A feature that is built on one or more walls of the pool to let the water overflow to another container. This gives the appearance of water extending to the horizon and self-cleans the surface of the pool of debris floating on the surface.

NSF: National Sanitation Foundation.

NITROGEN: Forms chloramines when combined with chlorine. It can be found in bather wastes such as perspiration, suntan oil, and hair tonics.

NON-CHLORINE SHOCK: A granular form of potassium monopersulfate. This is an oxidizer that acts as a catalyst to activate sodium bromide and breaks up chloramines and bromamines but cannot kill algae.

ORGANIC: A naturally occurring material such as perspiration, urine, oils, and plant material including leaves and bark.

OTO: A method of testing for free available chlorine levels in pool or spa water. Not believed to be as accurate as DPD.

OXIDIZER: Chemicals that release chlorine are among the group of chemicals classified as "oxidizers." These chemicals are in the halogen family and also include peroxides and persulfates.

OZONATOR: A device that uses oxygen to make ozone that is delivered in a pool or spa.

OZONE: A molecule that contains three atoms of oxygen; a powerful sanitizer. Ozonators make this molecule through UV radiation or discharge generators.

PARTS PER MILLION (PPM): A measurement used to calculate the parts per million or pounds per million pounds of chemicals and compounds in pool or spa water. For example, alkalinity should be kept at 80 to 120 ppm, by weight and in relation to the water it is dissolved in.

PH: The scale of relative acidity or alkalinity to soil or water. This scale runs from 0.0 to 14.0, with 7.0 being neutral. Below 7.0 is acidic, and above 7.0 is alkaline or basic.

PH BOUNCE: The rapid spiking and fluctuations of pH.

POTASSIUM MONOPERSULFATE: See non-chlorine shock.

POLYMER: An algaecide or algaestat made up of repeating molecules. Primarily used for green algae.

PRECIPITATION: To come out of solution or to become insoluble through a chemical action. Material that is forced out of solution will settle, stain, or scale, or remain suspended in the water.

PRESSURE SWITCH: A switch that can be activated by pressure. It can work in the reverse way that if no pressure is exerted, leaving the device inactivated. It can also be used as a safety switch.

PRESSURE GAUGE: A device that shows the pressure of the water in a system. Usually mounted on the filter.

PRIMING: Starting a flow of water to the suction side of a pump as water flows to the pressure side of the pump. Suction is then increased until the limits of the pump have been met.

PSI: Pounds per square inch. The measurement of pressure on a unit.

PVC: Polyvinyl chloride. A plastic-like product that is used for pipes, fittings, and pieces of equipment. It is chemical- and sun-resistant and can handle a great deal of pressure. Has good strength for its weight.

QUATERNARY AMMONIUM COMPOUND: A type of algaestat composed of ammonia compounds. It is commonly called Quats.

RATE OF TURNOVER: The time that it takes to circulate the entire amount of water in a pool or spa.

REAGENT: The chemical indicator used to test water balance. This can be a liquid, powder, or tablet.

REFLEXOLOGY: A form of therapy that uses deep pressure applied to reflex points in the hands and feet.

RESIDUAL: Refers to free available chlorine levels that remain in the pool.

SANITIZER: A chemical agent used to oxidize bacteria.

SCALE: Mineral salts that are forced out of solution. A scaling condition is when deposits attach themselves to surfaces and fixtures in the pool. This can plug or restrict the flow of water if severe.

SEDIMENT: A solid material that has come out of solution in water.

SEQUESTERING AGENT: A chemical that locks up minerals so they stay in solution where the filter can take them out.

SERVICE FACTOR: A rating for the efficiency of an electric motor; 1 hp is equivalent to 746 watts of power.

SHOCK: See breakpoint chlorination.

SKIMMER: A device that skims the surface of the water for debris floating on the water's surface.

SLIDE VALVE: A valve that only has a filtration position and a backwash position.

SODA ASH: Sodium carbonate. Has a pH of 11.3 and reduces the acidic conditions of water. It is used to raise the pH in water.

SODIUM BICARBONATE: Baking soda. Has a pH of 8.3. Used to raise the alkalinity in a pool.

SODIUM BISULFATE: See dry acid.

SODIUM HYPOCHLORITE: Liquid chlorine used in pools. It has a pH of 12.95 and comes in different strengths. Liquid chlorine for pools averages 11.5 percent available chlorine. This element is very corrosive.

SODIUM TETRABORATE: Borax. Sodium tetraborate deca-hydrate is the product you buy in grocery stores while sodium tetraborate pentahydrate is used for pools. When dissolved in water, the two substances are identical. This is an EPA-approved algaestat under the name of ProTeam® Supreme. Can also be used to raise pH without affecting alkalinity.

SODIUM DICHLOR: A granular form of stabilized chlorine. Used in super-chlorination.

SOFT WATER: Water that has a low calcium and/or magnesium content.

SOLAR HEAT: The heating system on a pool or spa that absorbs the heat of the sun and ambient temperature to heat water by passing it through panels or chambers usually mounted on roofs.

SOLAR COVER: A cover that sits directly on top of the water of a spa or pool and resists the leakage of temperature and evaporation. Used with solar heat and with normal heating.

SPA WAND: A hand-operated vacuum that is designed to clean a spa. Usually utilizes a screen to filter the debris.

SPIKING: A term used to describe sudden changes in pH levels.

STABILIZER: See cyanuric acid.

STRAINER: The basket located inside the trap of a pump that removes larger debris before it enters the pump and the filter.

SUPER-CHLORINATION: Applying seven to ten times the normal amount of chlorine to the pool or spa water as an added boost for the removal of contaminants.

TANNINS: Polyphenols that destroy proteins and turn wood a darker color.

TEST STRIPS: Chemical reagent strips that accurately test water for various chemicals if an interference of a high chemical does not affect them.

THERMAE: The first form of man-made, large-scale spas that were used in Roman times.

TITRATION: A method used to test for total alkalinity, calcium hardness, and acid-base demand. After adding a certain titrate, the liquid reacts and changes colors.

TOTAL ALKALINITY: The buffering capacity of the water. Resists sudden changes or spikes in pH levels. Total alkalinity is the amount of alkaline substances that measure above a pH 7.0.

TOTAL DISSOLVED SOLIDS (TDS): A measure of all the matter that is dissolved in a solution. High TDS levels can oversaturate your water. TDS is removed by draining pool or spa water.

TRAP: Part of a pump that has a lid and a basket to trap large debris before it enters the pump and filter.

TURBIDITY: Cloudy, dull, hazy water.

VANISHING EDGE: See negative edge.

VENTURI: A part that is restricted in the center and open on the ends so when water is forced through it, the force of the water creates a vacuum. Usually found with older chlorine systems and ozone generators.

VERTICAL GRID FILTER: A filter made of independent grids with a coating of a special cloth.

WATER FEATURE: A design made out of rocks, a series of rocks, a waterfall, or any other design that is part of the pool that lets water flow over them to the pool for an unusual and enjoyable look.

WATSU: A form of body massage with warm water.

WEIR: A part that fits into a skimmer that is hinged or floats and regulates the amount of water that flows over the top of the object; only lets the debris on the top of the water enter for proper skimming. Also can be a floating weir, which is a cylinder-shaped object in a skimmer basket that also performs the same function.

WICKING: When wood absorbs water from the bottom side of the spa and pulls it up into the wood, similar to the way a wick in a kerosene lamp would do.

WINTERIZING: The process of getting a spa ready for winter months to prevent damage and freezing of the pool and equipment.

REFERENCES

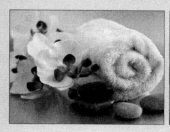 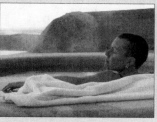 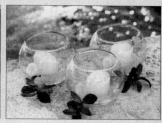

Important Contacts

Dan Hardy
Advance Aquatic Technologies, LLC
E-mail: poolandspabook@aol.com
www.bhpoolandspabook.com

Premium Leisure Spas
1-877-237-8772
E-mail: customerservice@premiumleisure.com
www.premiumleisure.com

Wooden Hot Tubs
SeaOtter WoodWorks, Inc
1-888-810-7717
www.woodentubs.com

Specialty Pools
Endless Pools
1-800-732-8660
www.endlesspools.com

Pool Supplies & Equipment (Online Sales)
Poolandspa.com
1-800-876-7647
E-mail: customerservice@poolandspa.com
www.poolandspa.com

BIBLIOGRAPHY

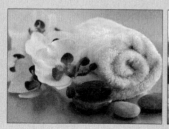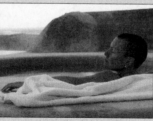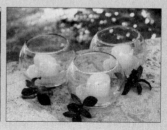

Avery, A. 1992. Aromatherapy and You. Kailua, HI: Blue Heron Hill Press.

Badia, P., et al. 1990. Responsiveness to olfactory stimuli presented in sleep. Physiology and Behavior 48: 87-90.

Edwards, L. 1994. Aromatherapy and essential oils. Healthy and Natural Journal, October, pp. 134-137.

Frawley, D. 1992. Herbs and the mind. In American Herbalism: Essays on Herbs and Herbalism, ed. by M. Tierra. Freedom, Calif.: Crossing Press.

Green, M. 1992. Simpler scents: The combined use of herbs and essential oils. In American Herbalism: Essays on Herbs and Herbalism, ed. by M. Tierra. Freedom, Calif.: Crossing Press.

Heinerman, J. 1988. Heinerman's Encyclopedia of Fruits, Vegetables, and Herbs. West Nyack, N.Y.: Parker Publishing.

Hillyer, P. 1994. "Making $cents with Aromatherapy." Whole Foods, February, pp. 26-35.

Hoffmann, D. 1987. Aromatherapy. In The Herbal Handbook. Rochester, Vt.: Healing Arts Press.

Kikuchi, A., et al. 1992. Effects of odors on cardiac response patterns and subjective states in a reaction time task. Psychologica Folia 51: 74-82.

Klemm, W. R., et al. 1992. Topographical EEG maps of human response to odors. Chemical Senses 17: 347-361.

Lavabre, M. 1990. Aromatherapy Workbook. Rochester, Vt.: Healing Arts Press.

Ludvigson, H., and T. Rottman. 1989. Effects of ambient odors of lavender and cloves on cognition, memory, affect and mood. Chemical Sense 14: 525-536.

Nakano, Y., et al. 1992. A study of fragrance impressions, evaluation and categorization. Psychologica Folia 51: 83-90.

Price, S. 1991. Aromatherapy for Common Ailments. New York: Simon and Schuster.

Raphael, A. 1994. "Ahh! Aromatherapy." Delicious, December pp. 47-48.

Roberts, A., and J. Williams. 1992. The effect of olfactory stimulation on fluency, vividness of imagery and associated mood: A preliminary study. British Journal of Medical Psychology 65: 197-199.

Rose, J. 1988. Healing scents from herbs: Aromatherapy. In Herbal Handbook. Escondido, Calif.: Bernard Jensen Enterprises.

Smith, D. G., et al. 1992. Verbal memory elicited by ambient odor. Perceptual and Motor Skills 74: 339-343.

Tisserand, M. 1988. Aromatherapy for Women. Rochester, Vt.: Healing Arts Press.

Tsuchiya, T., et al. 1991. Effects of olfactory stimulation on the sleep time induced by pentobarbital administration in mice. Brain Research Bulletin 26: 397-401.

Valnet, J. 1982. The Practice of Aromatherapy. London: C. W. Daniel.

MedicineNet: **www.medicinenet.com**

American Cancer Society: **www.cancer.org/docroot/ETO/content/ETO_5_3x_Hydrotherapy.asp**

National Center for Biotechnology Information: **www.ncbi.nlm.nih.gov/pmc/articles/PMC1297510**

The Association of Pool and Spa Professionals: **www.apsp.org/clientresources/documents/sensiblewayspahottub_lores_jul06.pdf**

Extreme Spa Covers: **www.extreme-spa-covers.com/spa_covers_features.htm**

Environmental Protection Agency — Air Quality Awareness: **www.epa.gov/airnow/airaware/day1-ozone.html**

BIBLIOGRAPHY

Hot Tub Essentials: **www.hottubessentials.com/ozone_FAQs. htm**

Castaway Pools & Spas: **www.castawaypools.com/faqs.htm**

The Physics Hypertextbook: **http://physics.info/convection**

eMedicine from WebMD: **http://emedicine.medscape.com/ article/324974-overview**

Swimming Pools Etc.: **www.swimmingpoolsetc.com/spa-parts-air-buttons.htm**

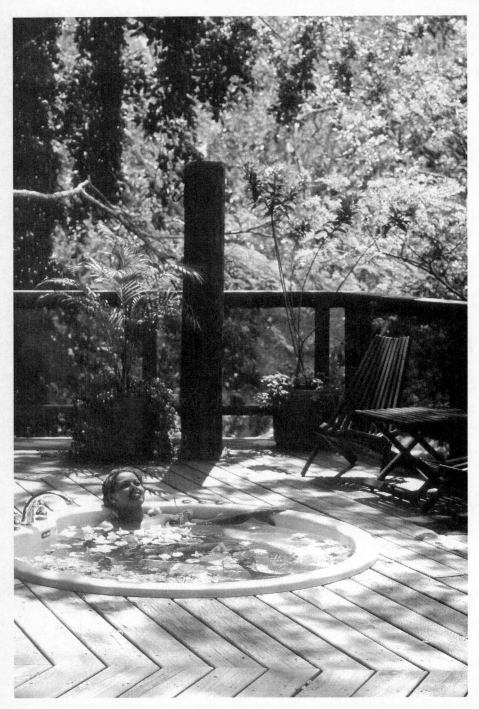

AUTHOR BIOGRAPHY

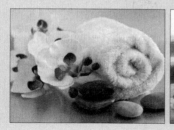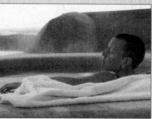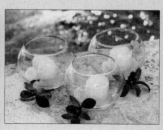

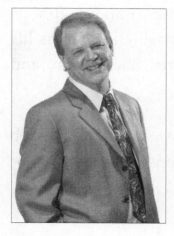

Dan Hardy was born August 16, 1953, in Hereford, Texas. His background in pool maintenance began on his dad's country club in Clovis, New Mexico, in 1976. Ten years later, he opened his own business delivering and setting up spas and doing pool work along with installing in-ground foundations for manufactured homes in Albuquerque, New Mexico.

He moved to Ocala, Florida, in 1998 and opened Dan's Perfect Pool Service, Pool Palace, Mount View Enterprises, LLC, and then D & C Enterprises. In 2007, he could not resist the chance to re-open another service company. He has worked on many fabulous pools for celebrities in Ocala, including John Travolta and Kelly Preston; Terri Jones-Thayer, former

Miss World and Revlon®'s perfect "Charlie Girl;" and Brock Marion, a former Dallas Cowboy.

Dan graduated from Boys Ranch High School in Texas in 1971, and from General Motors Technical School in Oklahoma City, Oklahoma, in 1972. He attended Amarillo College for auto mechanics and studied mechanical engineering at Tacoma Community College in Washington. Besides a career as a pool professional, Dan is a licensed Realtor® in Florida and a partner with his wife, Carol, in real estate for a local brokerage. He has two daughters, Randi and Marcie, and two sons, Matthew and Michael. His pride is his grandkids: Austin Shane, Kenzy Marie, Shelby Lyn, and Seth Randall.

For those needing assistance, Dan has a page on his Web site, **www.bhpoolandspabook.com,** to answer questions for people who have purchased this book.

INDEX

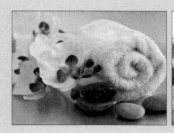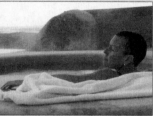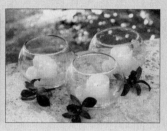